AF901457

Pet Owner Educational Atlas

DOGS

SERVET

Plaza Antonio Beltrán Martínez nº 1, planta 8 - letra I
(Centro empresarial El Trovador)
50002 Zaragoza - Spain

First printing: 2014

This book was originally published in Spanish under the title:
Atlas de información al propietario. Especie canina
© 2014 Grupo Asís Biomedia, SL
ISBN Spanish edition: 978-84-941975-9-8

Translation:
Óscar Deza del Olmo

Illustrators:
Jacob Gragera Artal
Paula Marco Peinado

ISBN: 978-84-942775-3-5
DL: Z 880-2014

Design, layout and printing:
Servet editorial - Grupo Asís Biomedia, SL
www.grupoasis.com
info@grupoasis.com

GRUPO asis

Servet is the publishing house of Grupo Asís

PROLOGUE

When Servet contacted me to collaborate in the development of *Pet owner educational atlas. Dogs*, I remembered a very basic book but with the same practical idea we used in the first clinic where I was trained. It was helpful to explain the disease to our clients, and they appreciated it and showed a great interest. I always thought that really did it "egotistically" as to the extent that owners understand what happens to their pets, it would help to explain the symptoms, evolution and keys that will help their diagnosis and treatment. It is essential to the work of veterinary surgeons.

The result of this collaboration is a simple work, but with a thorough work of visual and technical collection. Make things easy is the hardest.

Currently, the accurate information supported by images turns into the ideal way of communication between the veterinarian and the client. In this sense, we must acknowledge the great work done by illustrators Jacob Gragera and Paula Marco. They have caught the keys of each pathology through attractive schemes and images that clarify Tatiana Blasco's and Óscar Deza's texts, without forgetting the design and layout done by Marian Izaguerri.

But we are not facing a uniquely informative work. The technical level of the contents allows the veterinary surgeon to explain general concepts of the main dog diseases, some advanced and always updated. I was pleasantly surprised that outbreak data reported a few months ago in France and Spain were included in the sheet dedicated to rabies.

Working with Servet team in the review of the book has been a pleasure. We all want the pages and binding are worn down quickly, which means that the atlas is fulfilling its task in the hands of veterinary surgeons.

Alberto Barneto Carmona

Ayavet Veterinary Clinic

Boadilla del Monte, Madrid

alberto.barneto@ayavet.com

Table of contents

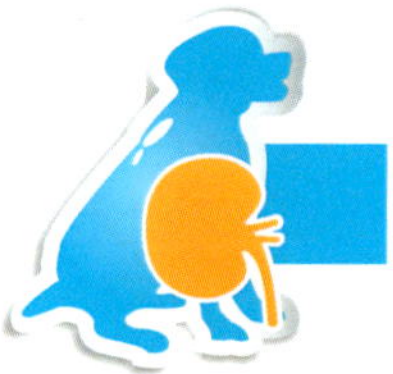

01 ANATOMY AND PHYSIOLOGY

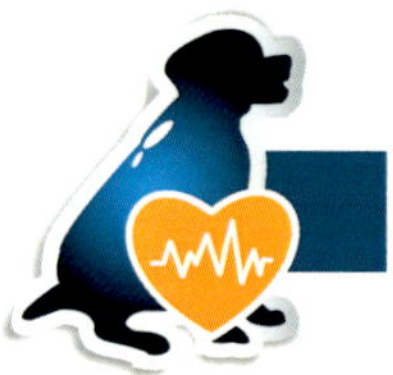

02 MAIN CONDITIONS BY SYSTEM

Musculoskeletal system

Urogenital system

Cardiorespiratory system

Endocrine system

Skin and adnexa

Digestive system

Eyes

Nervous system

03 INFECTIOUS DISEASES

04 SPECIAL TECHNIQUES

05 BEHAVIOUR AND MANAGEMENT

1 Dog skeleton

Fibrous, cartilaginous and synovial joints

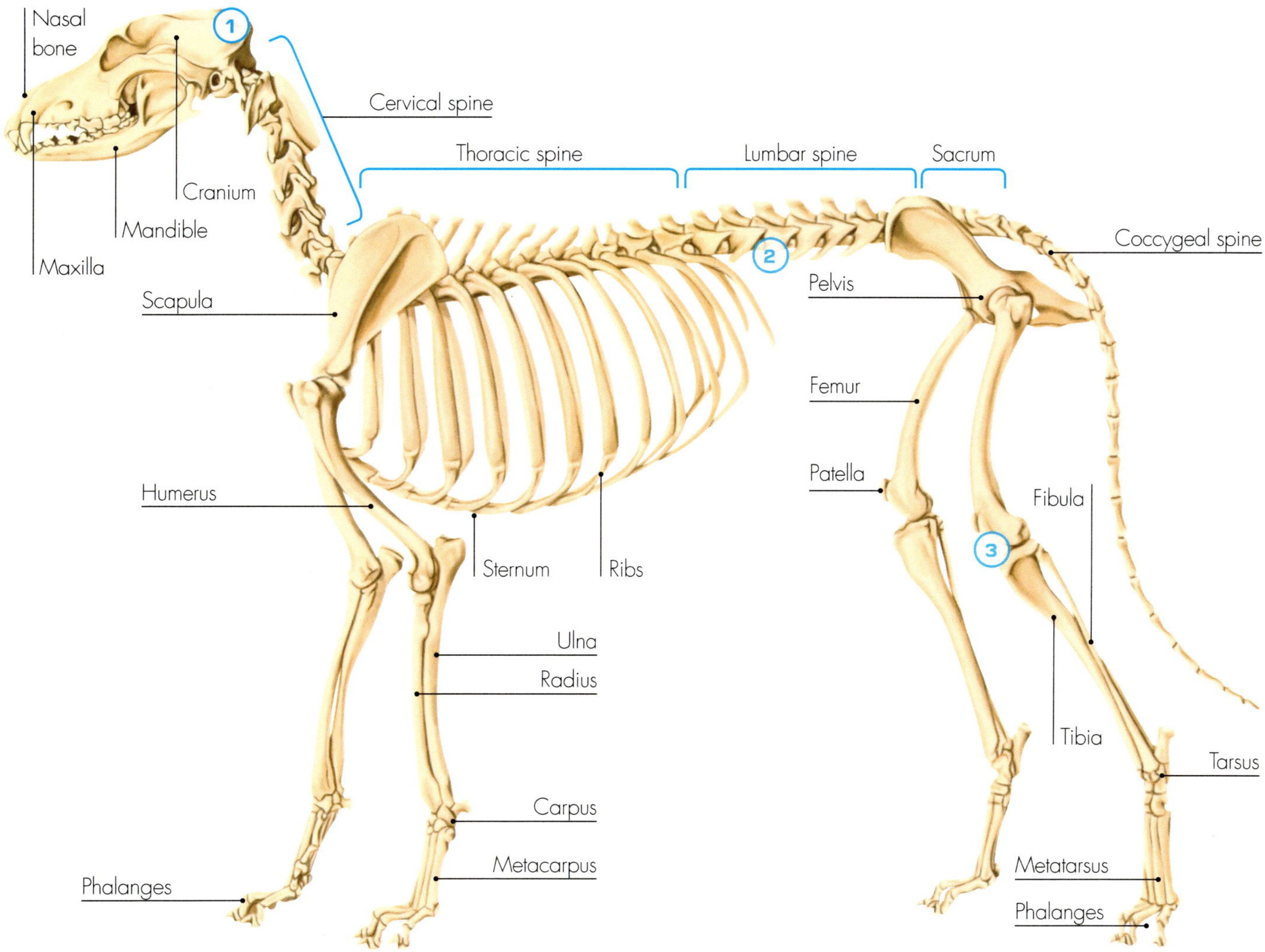

1 FIBROUS JOINT
(cranial sutures)

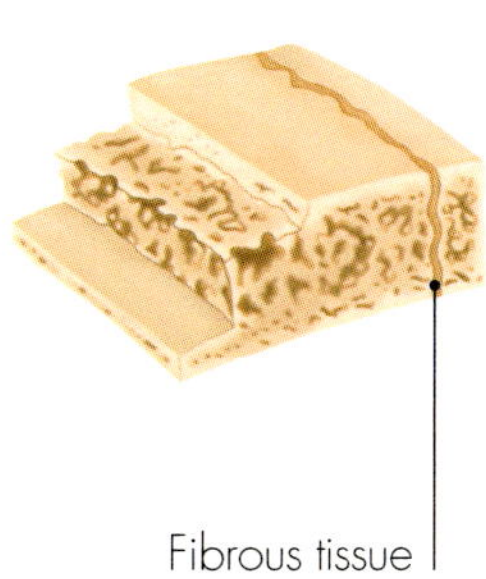

2 CARTILAGINOUS JOINT
(intervertebral joints)

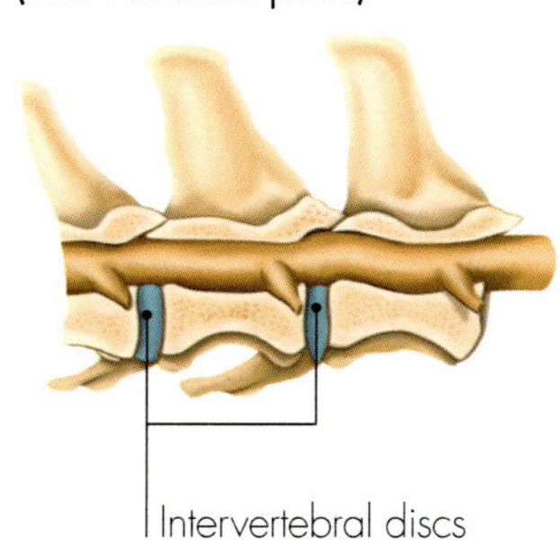

3 SYNOVIAL JOINT
(stifle, elbow, shoulder, hip, etc.)

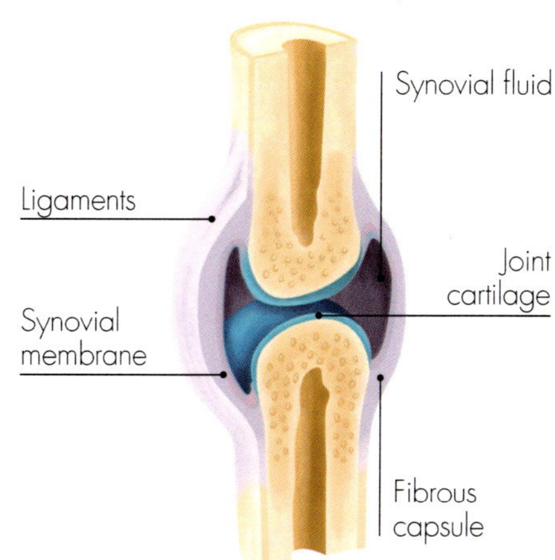

2 Dog muscles

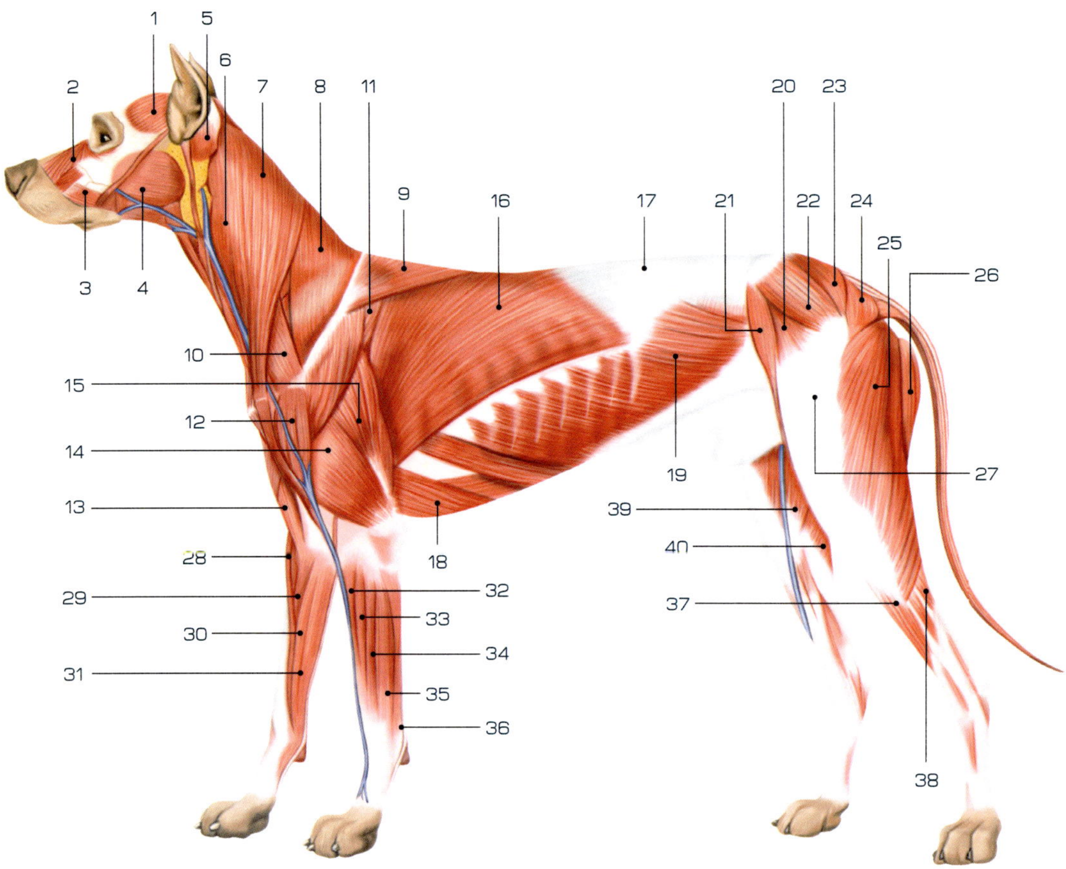

1. Temporal muscle
2. Levator nasolabialis muscle
3. Orbicularis oris muscle
4. Masseter muscle
5. Auricularis muscles
6. Sternocephalic muscle
7. Brachiocephalic muscle
8. Trapezius muscle, cervical part
9. Trapezius muscle, thoracic part
10. Omotransversarius muscle
11. Infraspinatus muscle
12. Deltoid muscle
13. Triceps brachii muscle
14. Triceps brachii muscle, lateral head
15. Triceps brachii muscle, long head
16. Latissimus dorsi muscle
17. Lumbar fascia
18. Deep pectoral muscle
19. Abdominal external oblique muscle
20. Tensor fasciae latae muscle
21. Sartorius muscle
22. Gluteus medius muscle
23. Gluteus superficialis muscle
24. Coccygeal muscle
25. Biceps femoris muscle
26. Semitendinosus muscle
27. Fascia lata
28. Brachioradialis muscle
29. Pronator teres muscle
30. Flexor carpi radialis muscle
31. Superficial digital flexor muscle
32. Extensor carpi radialis muscle
33. Extensor digitorum communis muscle
34. Extensor digitorum lateralis muscle
35. Extensor carpi ulnaris muscle
36. Flexor carpi ulnaris muscle
37. Tibialis cranialis muscle
38. Gastrocnemius muscle
39. Gracilis muscle
40. Semimembranosus muscle

Muscles of the abdomen

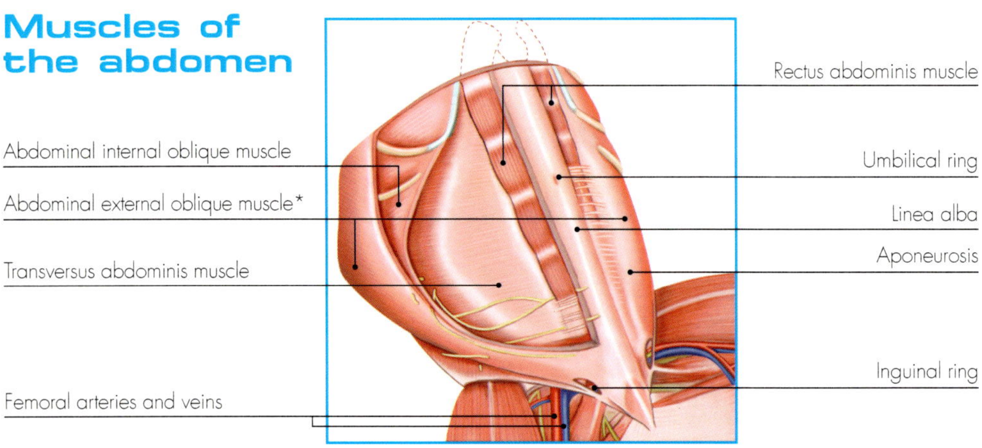

*Removed in the left side of the drawing to show the deeper muscles.

MUSCULOSKELETAL

3 Joint osteochondrosis

Shoulder and stifle

Osteochondrosis affects the developmental period (4-9 months), usually large breeds and rapid growth. It can occur in almost any joint, but the shoulder, stifle and elbow highlight due its clinical importance (see next slide).

It is twice more frequent in males than in females.

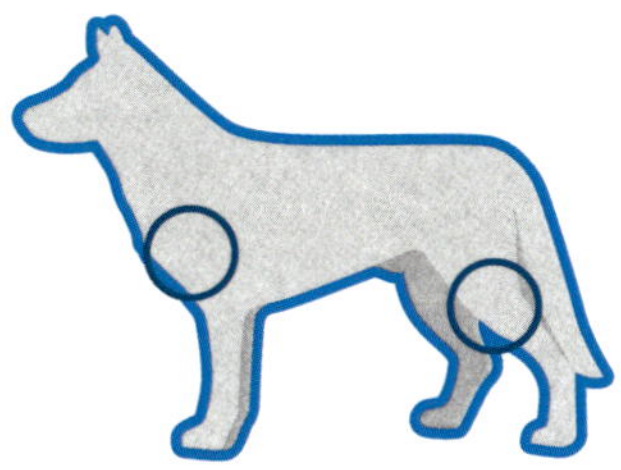

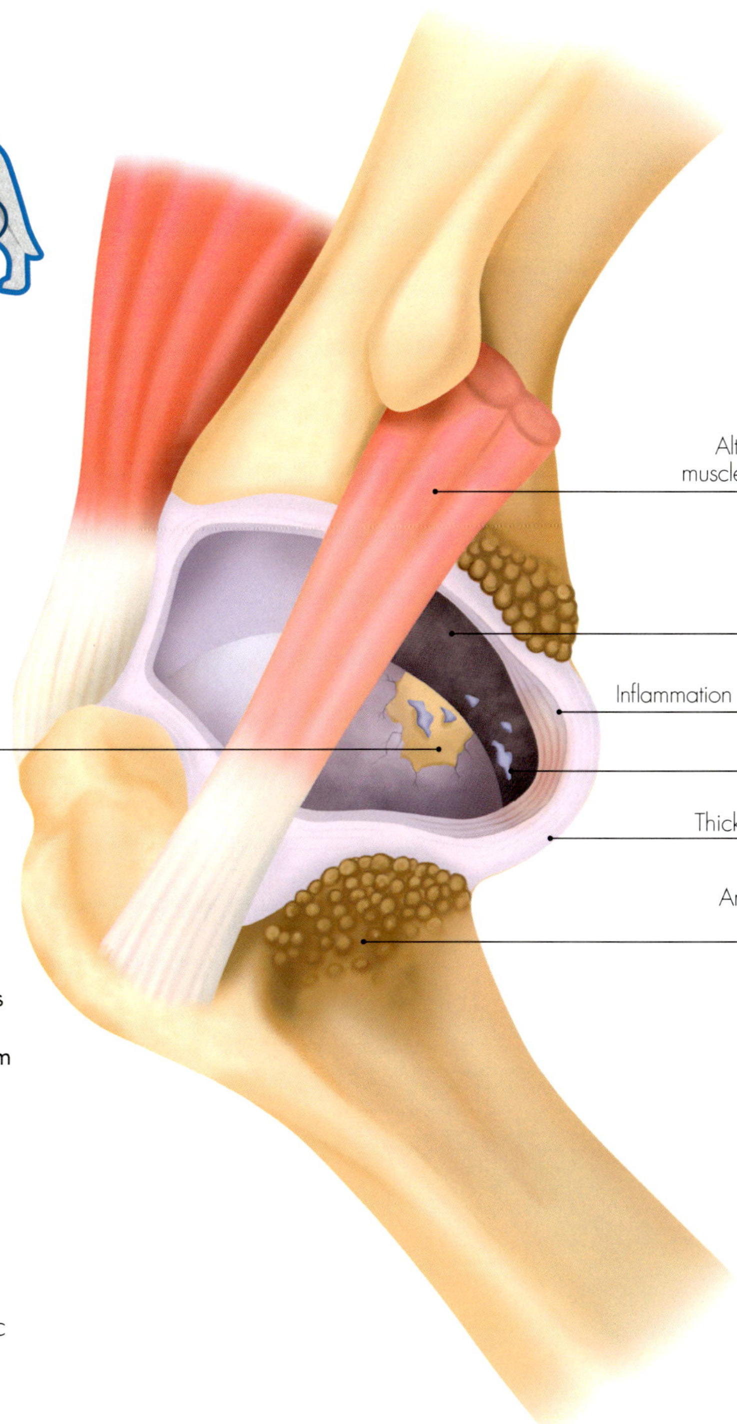

Osteochondritis / osis dissecans (OCD): when a portion of the affected cartilage separates from the joint surface and is loose, forming a "joint mouse".

Risk factors

- Direct: rapid growth and trauma.
- Indirect: nutrition, hormones, genetic predisposition and size.

MUSCULOSKELETAL

4 Elbow dysplasia

Genetic developmental disease, polygenic nature, which can be given either unilaterally or bilaterally. It is more frequent in large breeds and males are more affected than females.

One or more of these causes can be combined

- Osteochondritis dissecans.
- Ununited anconeal process.
- Fragmented coronoid process.
- Humeroradial and humeroulnar incongruence.

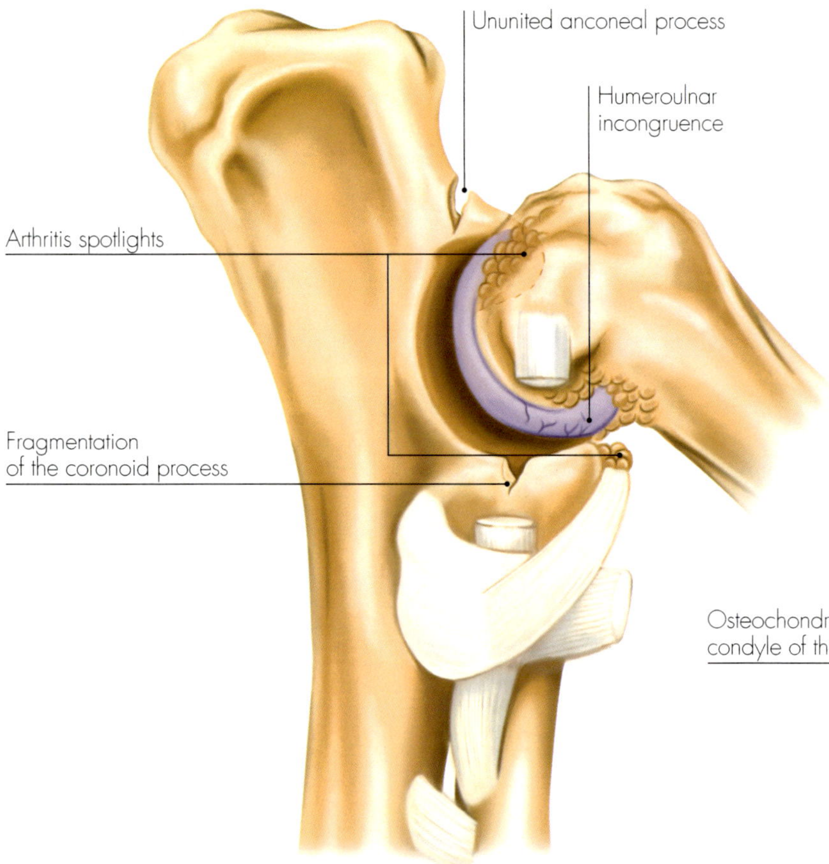

MEDIAL VIEW

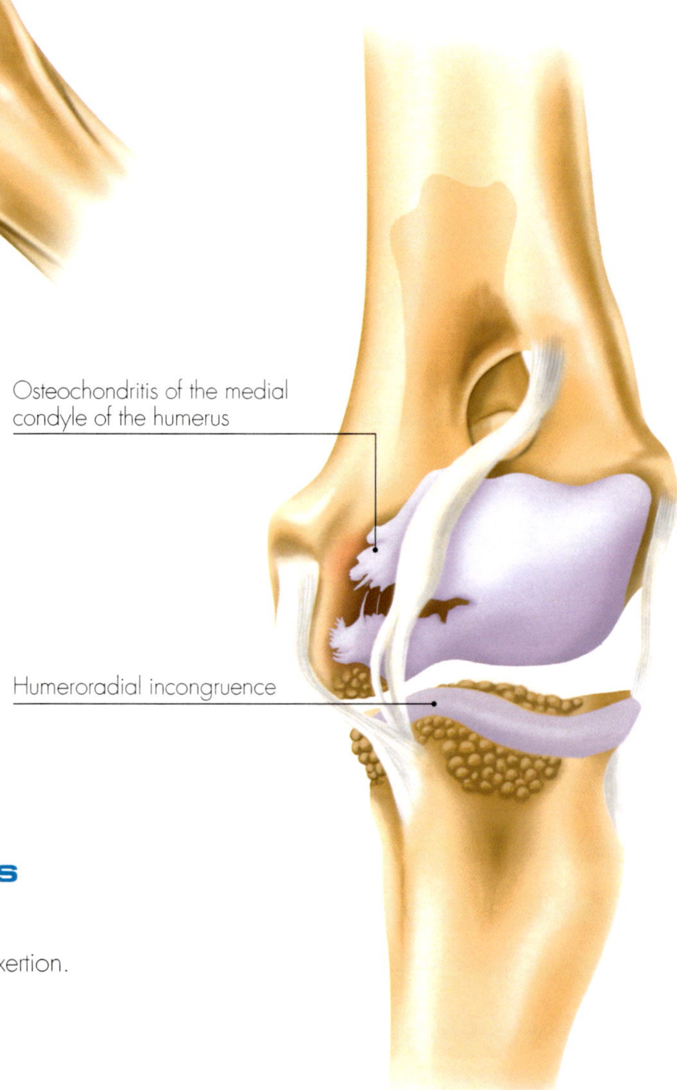

ANTERIOR VIEW

Early symptoms may occur within 4-5 months with lameness and intolerance to exercise.

Risk factors

- Incorrect feeding.
- Overweight or overexertion.
- Trauma.

Medical / surgical treatment

- Using medical or surgical treatment depends on the degree of dysplasia.
- Resolution by arthroscopic techniques provides good results.

MUSCULOSKELETAL

5 Hip dysplasia

It is the most frequent congenital osteoarticular disease in dogs, typical of large and medium breeds. It is accompanied by joint degenerative changes (osteoarthrosis), causing inflammation and pain, which produces muscle atrophy due to disuse. In puppies, it is usually detected at 5-6 months with radiographs.

Aetiology

Multifactorial, including both hereditary and environmental factors:

- Rapid growth.
- Excessive nutritional intake.
- Mild and repeated trauma.

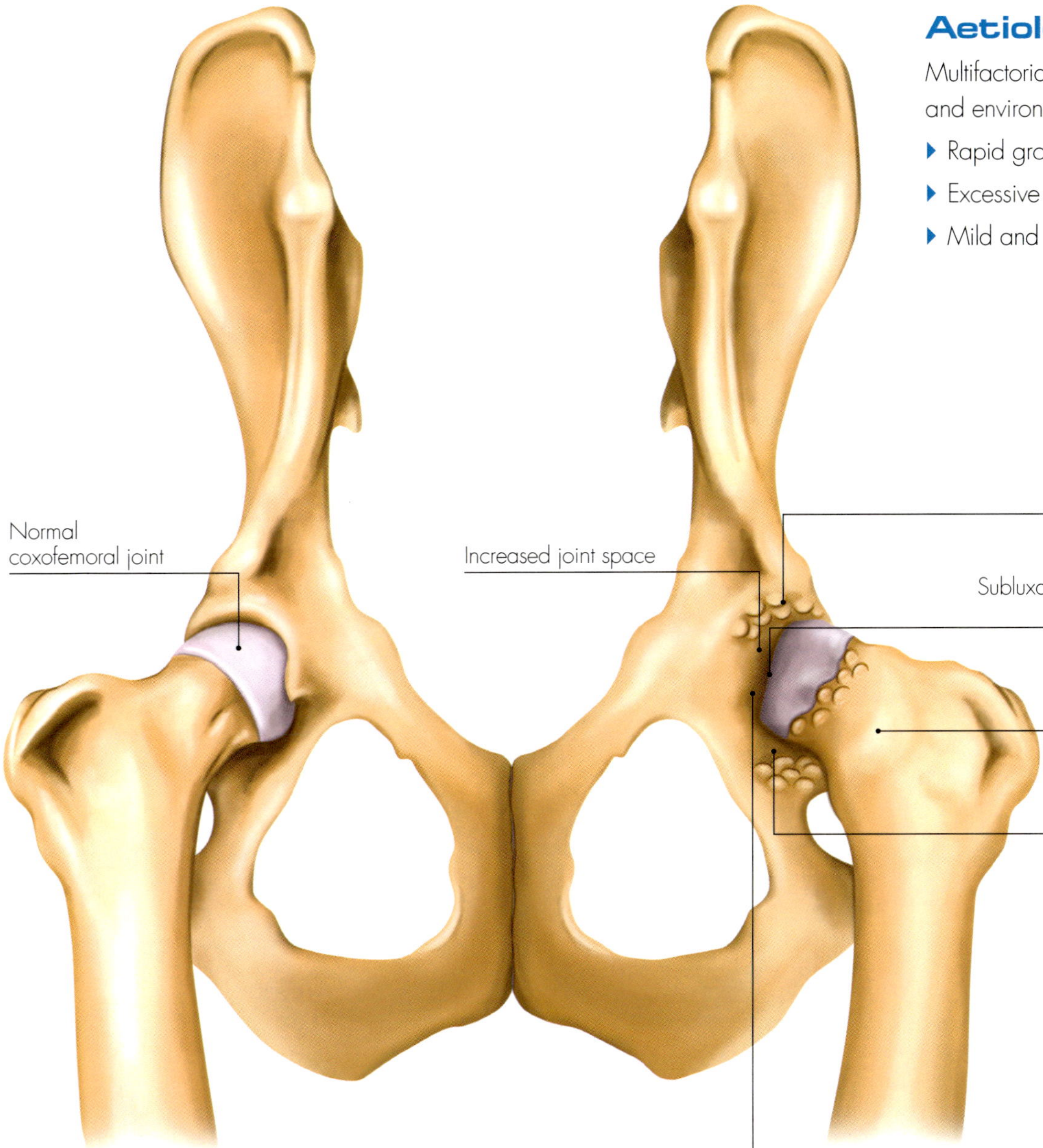

Surgical / medical treatment

In severe cases, it can be treated by surgery and provided with supportive therapy (anti-inflammatory, cartilage protective, moderate exercise, etc.).

The observed symptoms may not be directly related to the alterations detected in the radiograph (dogs with dysplasia and very little pain or dogs with little dysplasia and severe pain).

MUSCULOSKELETAL

6 Vertebral disorders

Spondyloarthrosis, herniation and luxation

Most commonly affected regions:

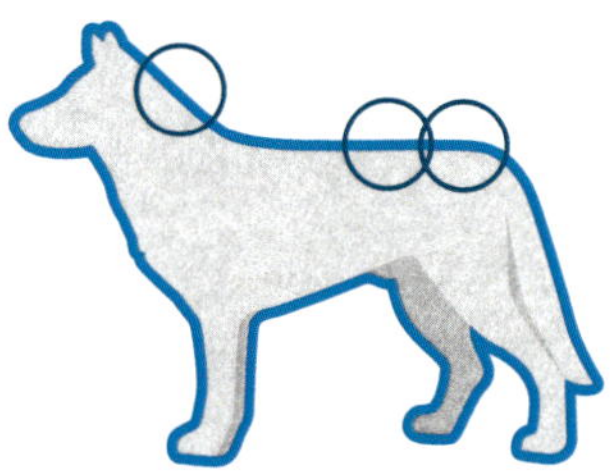

Cervical, thoracolumbar and lumbosacral (cauda equina syndrome).

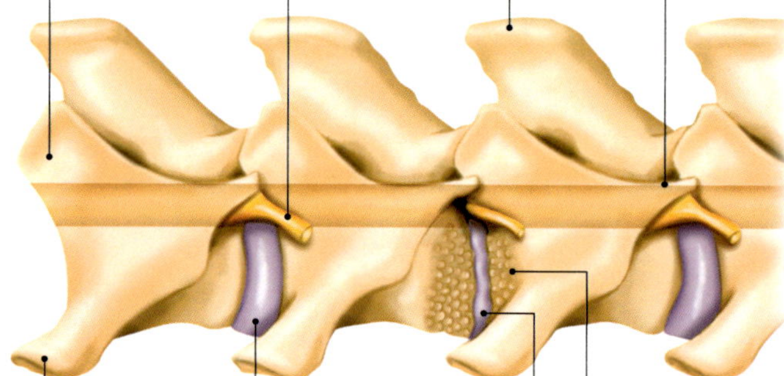

SPONDYLOARTHROSIS

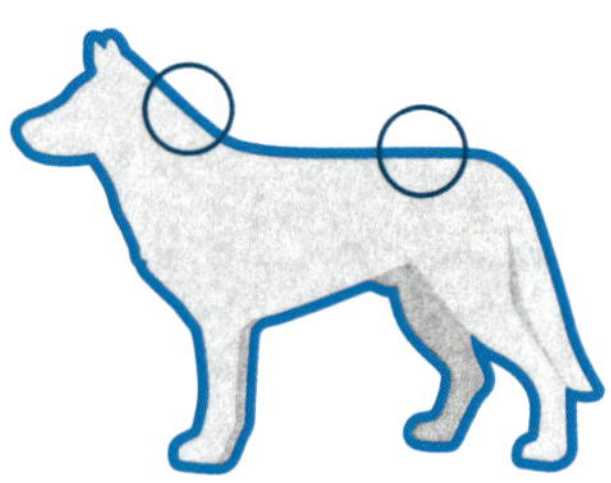

Cervical and thoracolumbar.

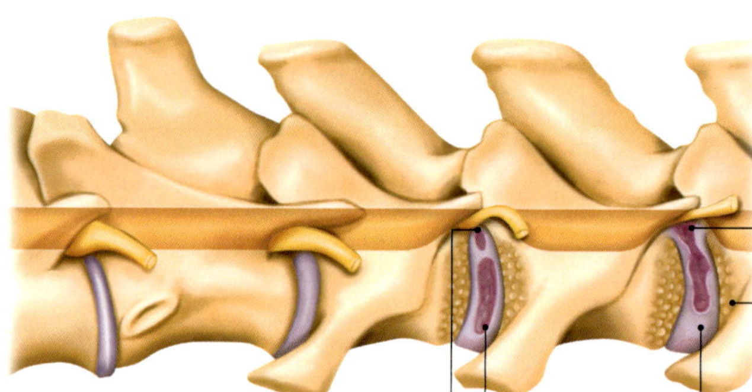

INTERVERTEBRAL DISC HERNIATION

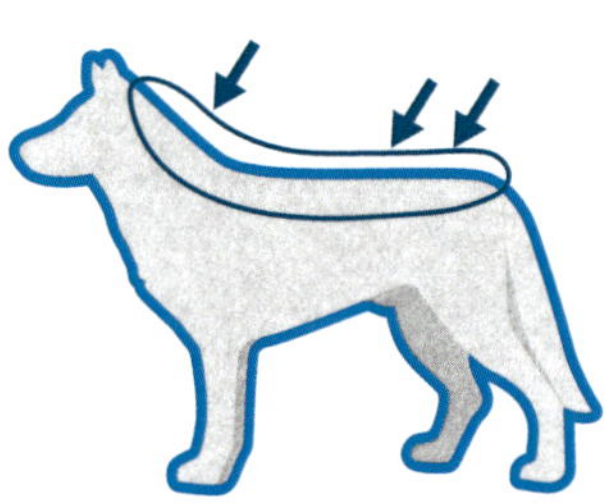

It can be seen in any vertebrae but it is more frequent in the cervical, thoracolumbar and lumbosacral regions.

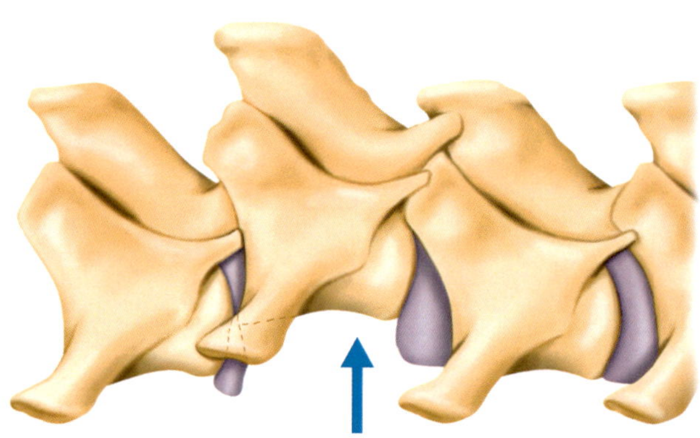

VERTEBRAL LUXATION

- Often associated with severe trauma (accidents, violent blows, etc.).
- It is recommended to investigate other lesions by radiographs of the whole body.

Consequences of spinal cord compression

- Pain (antalgic postures).
- Incoordination.
- Paresis or paralysis of the limbs.
- Loss of sensitivity.
- Urination and defecation problems (incontinence or retention).

MUSCULOSKELETAL

7 Avascular necrosis of the femoral head

Legg-Calvé-Perthes disease

Bone disease that mainly affects small and toy breeds. It occurs in young dogs (4-12 months old) and it is usually unilateral (85 % of cases).

Clinical signs

- Pain.
- Lack of support or immobilization.
- Muscular atrophy of the affected limb.

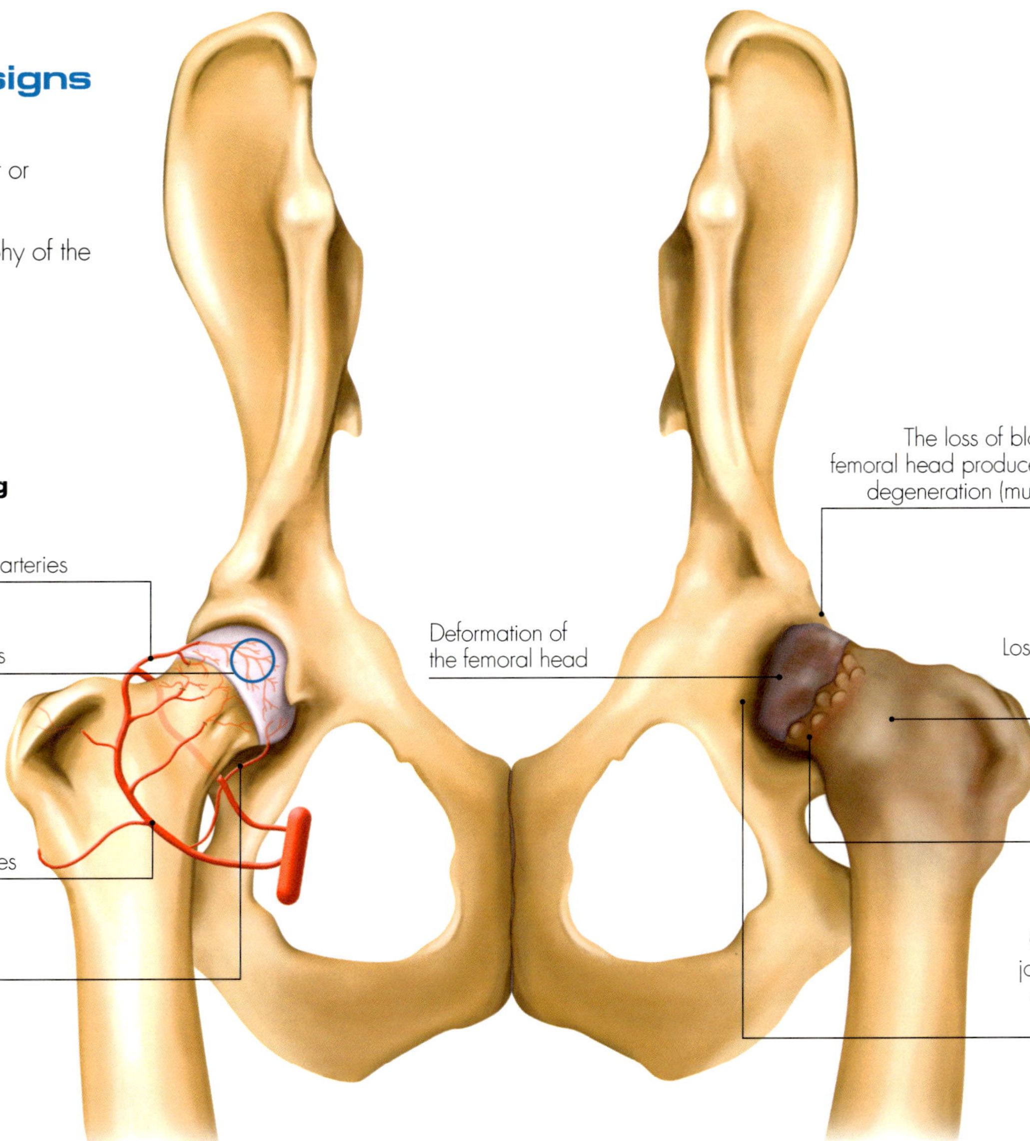

Surgical treatment

Removing the femoral head if physiotherapy and rehabilitation techniques do not work after 4 weeks.

Predisposing factors

- Breed (small and toy breeds).
- Congenital.
- Environmental (difficult births).
- Developmental disorders (disproportionate growth).
- Trauma (producing ischaemia repeatedly).

MUSCULOSKELETAL

8 Rupture of the anterior cruciate ligament (RACL)

It is one of the most common musculoskeletal conditions in the dog. It mainly affects large dogs (>20 kg) and certain breeds (Newfoundland, Labrador and Golden Retriever, Mastiff, Rottweiler, etc.).

It is the most frequent cause of secondary degenerative osteoarthritis in the stifle.

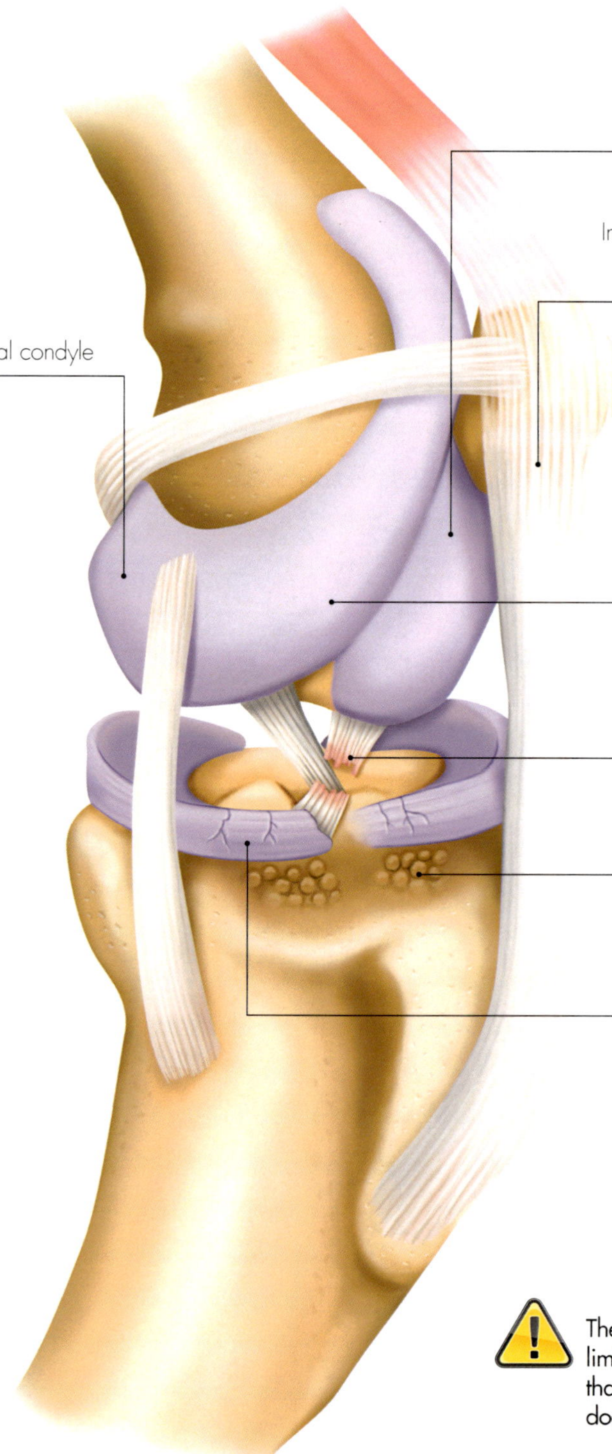

Risk factors

- Obesity and physical inactivity.
- Muscular atrophies.
- Degenerative joint diseases.

Diagnosis

- Acute lameness with lack of support or just support of fingers.
- Palpation and drawer and cranial tibial compression tests.
- Confirmation by radiography, magnetic resonance imaging, arthroscopy, arthrotomy or synovial fluid analysis.

Surgical treatment

It can be solved by surgical techniques:

- Extracapsular.
- Intracapsular.
- Modifying the stifle biomechanics.

The ligament of the opposite limb can be broken in less than 2 years in 30-40 % of dogs which suffer RACL.

UROGENITAL

9 Acute and chronic kidney disease

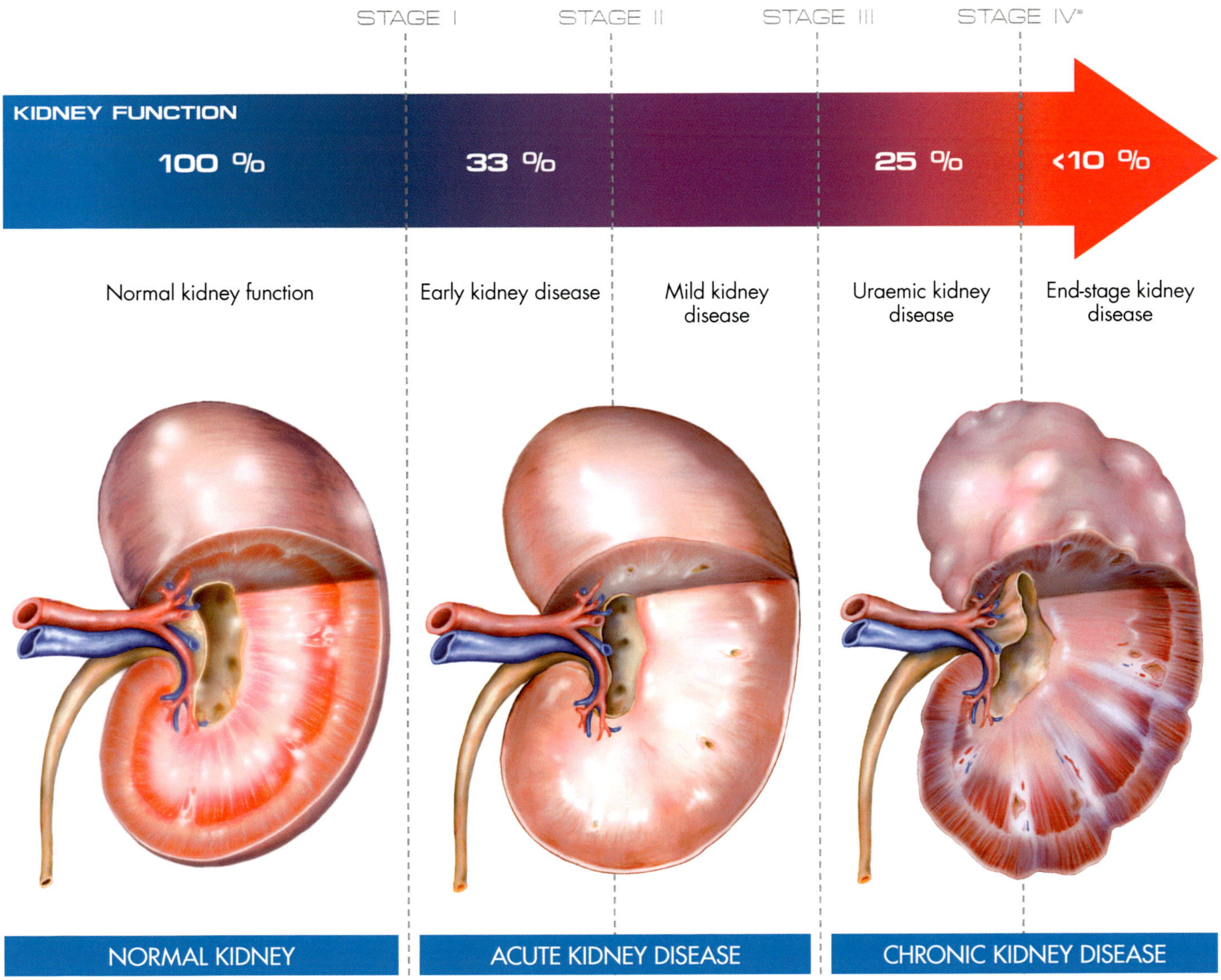

Diagnosis

Early diagnosis is essential:

- Clinical history and complete physical examination.
- Urea and creatinine, calcium and phosphorus and other blood tests.
- Urinalysis.
- Arterial pressure.
- Radiograph, ultrasound scan.
- Biopsy.

*Classification accepted by the International Renal Interest Society (IRIS).

Medical treatment

Key points of the treatment of acute kidney disease:

- Reversing the cause and avoiding risk factors.
- Correcting uraemia and water, electrolyte and acid-base imbalances.
- Regaining normal urine elimination.
- Individualised drug treatment for each case.

Dietary treatment

Nutritional support with appropriate diets.

UROGENITAL

10 Urinary calculi

Urethral obstruction

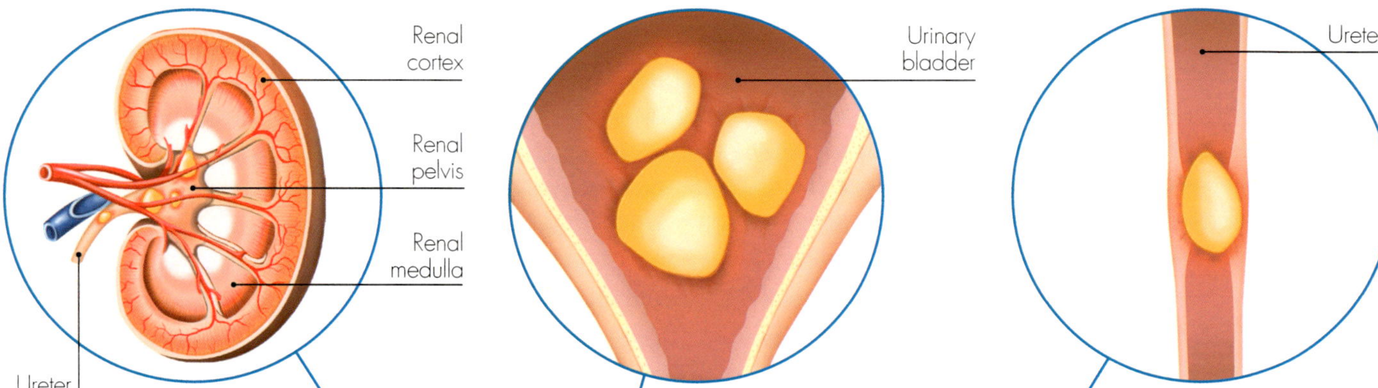

Calculi formation in the renal pelvis (nephroliths)

Calculi formation in the urinary bladder

Calculi can pass into the ureter and cause an obstruction

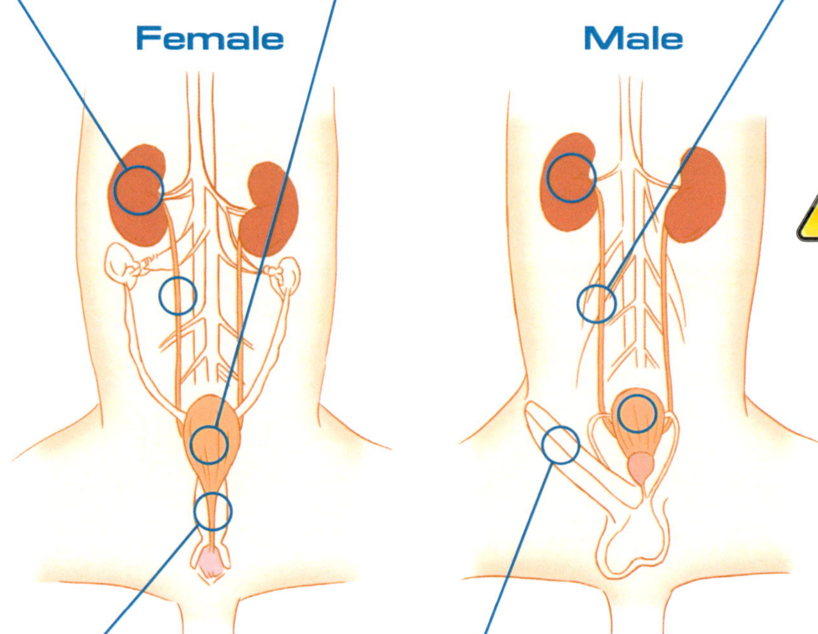

Females often have fewer problems with urinary calculi obstruction because of the anatomical conformation of the urethra, whose path is shorter and wider.

The path of the adjacent urethra is a frequent place for urethral obstruction by calculi due to the presence of the baculum in the male.

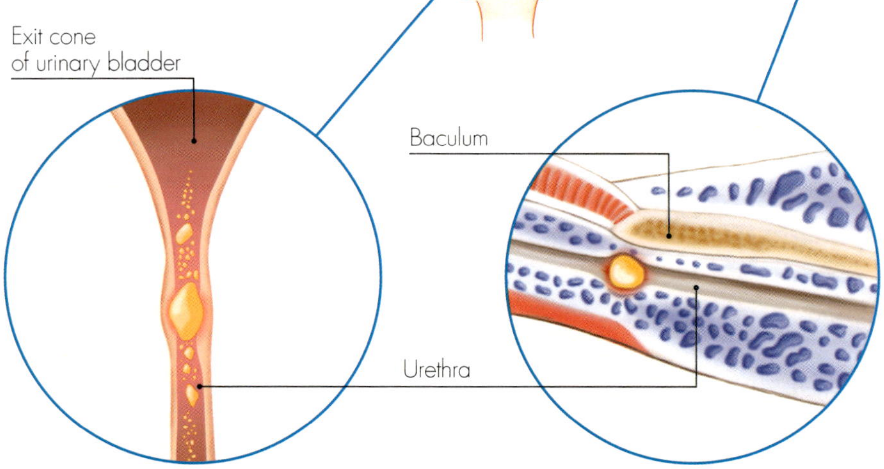

Calculi may pass into the urethra and cause an obstruction

TYPES OF URINARY CRYSTALS

Alkaline urine

- Magnesium ammonium phosphate (struvite)
- Ammonium biurate (also in acid urine)
- Calcium carbonate (rarely)

Acid urine

- Calcium oxalate
- Amorphous urates
- Bilirubin

Amino acid crystals

- Cystine
- Tyrosine

URoGENITAL

11 The oestrus cycle of the bitch

The sexual cycle of the bitch is monoestrous, spontaneous ovulation and usually has two oestrous cycles per year. Each cycle is divided into 4 phases: anoestrus, pro-oestrus, oestrus and dioestrus.

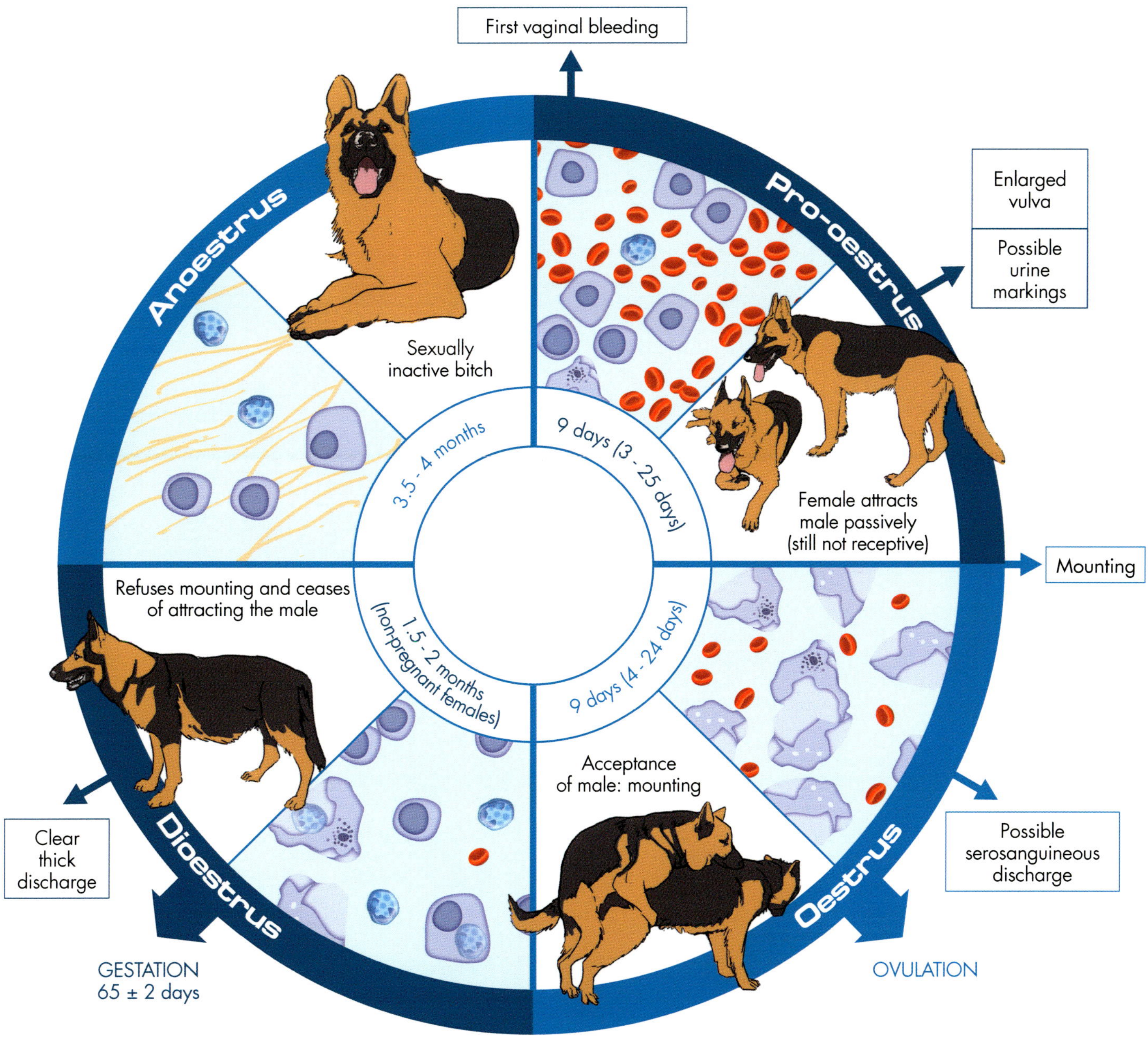

COMPONENTS OF THE VAGINAL CYTOLOGY PERFORMED TO DETERMINE THE CYCLE PHASES

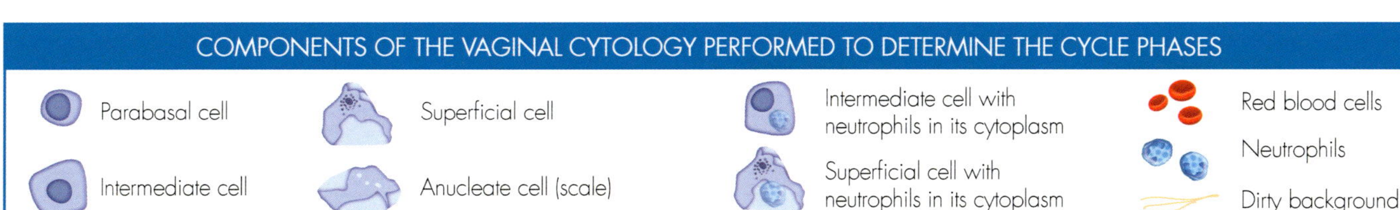

UROGENITAL

12 Neutering in males and females

Ovariohysterectomy — Female

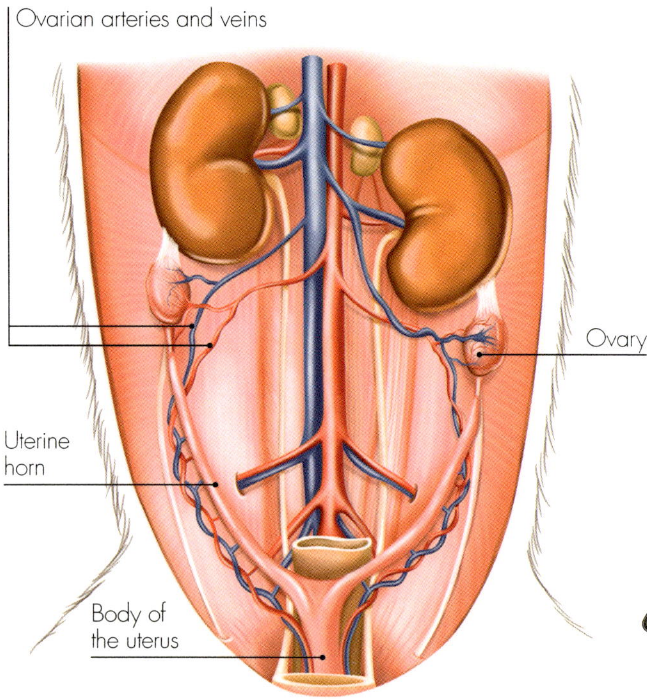

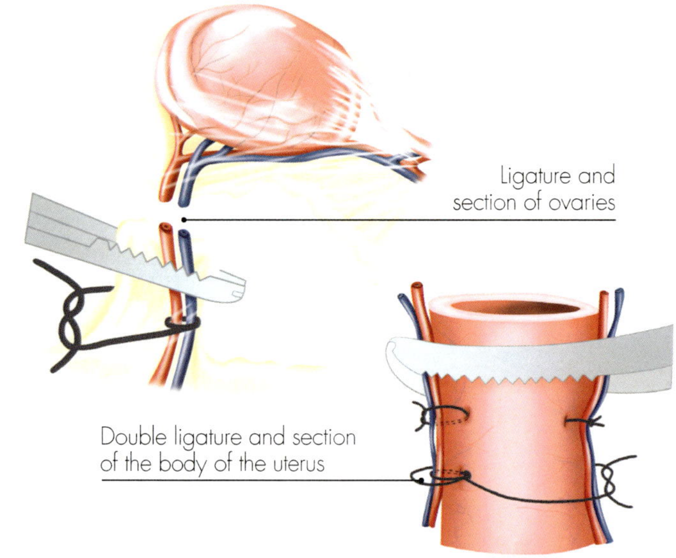

The risk of mammary tumours is reduced if ovariohysterectomy is done before 2.5 years of age. It also prevents ovarian neoplasia, vaginal hyperplasia, vaginal prolapse, cystic endometrial hyperplasia and pyometra.

Vasectomy / orchiectomy — Male

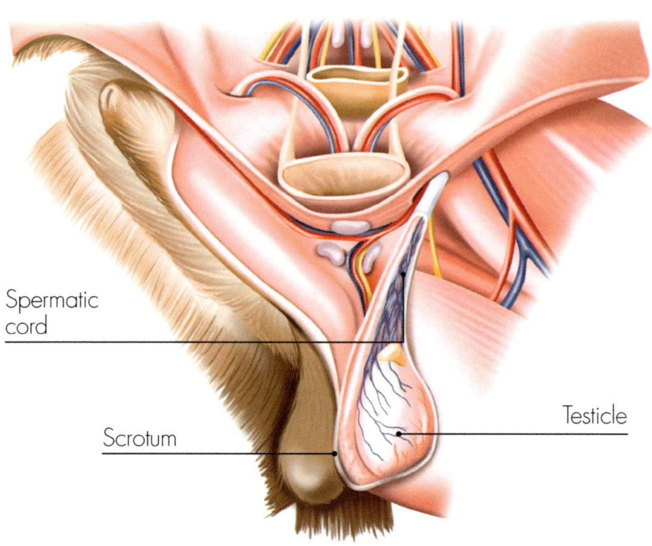

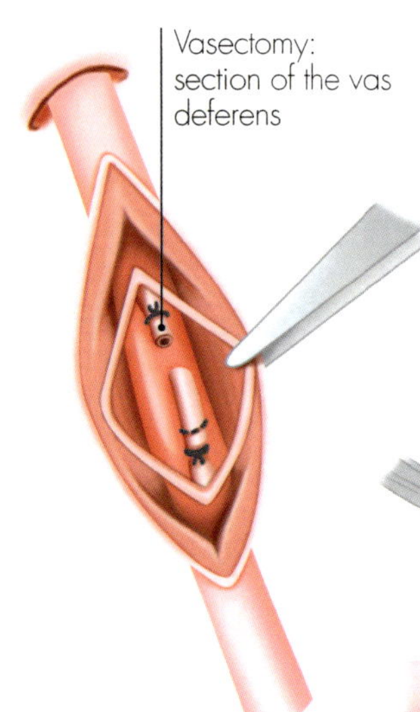

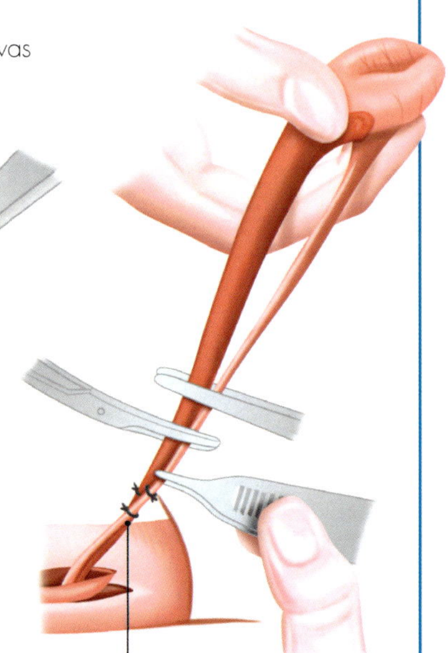

Males can also be pharmacologically neutered by subcutaneous implants or injectable treatments which inhibit the hormonal activity and sperm production.

Mating must be avoided for 3 weeks after vasectomy, as there are sperm at the end of the vas deferens.

Orchiectomy: surgical removal of the testicles

UROGENITAL

13 Most frequent types of dystocia in dogs

Dystocia is defined as difficulty or inability to expel the foetus from the uterus through the birth canal. It may be due to problems in the mother (75 %) or foetus (25 %). In brachycephalic or toy breeds almost 100 % of births are dystocic.

Maternal dystocia

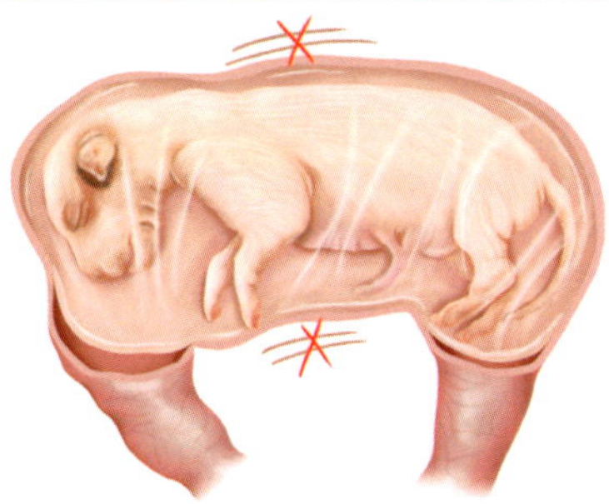
Uterine inertia

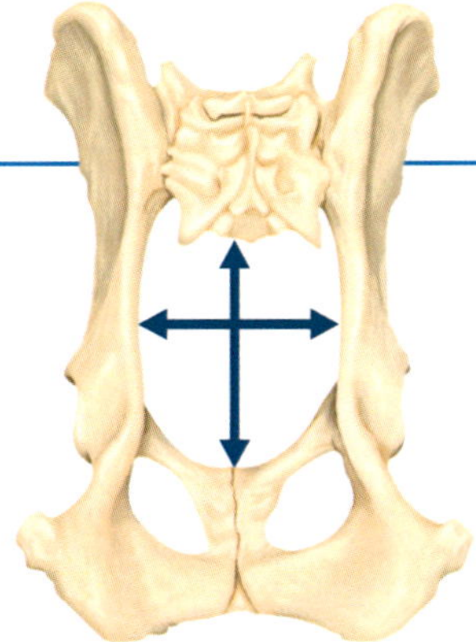
Narrowing of the pelvic canal

Types of dystocia

Maternal

- Uterine inertia (lack of contractions).
- Narrowing of the pelvic canal.
- Stenosis of the vagina.
- Hormonal disorders.
- Structural anomalies.

Foetal

- Abnormal presentations: bent forelegs, lateral or backward bending of the head, etc.
- Excessive size of the foetus.
- Malformations.
- Foetal death.

Assisted natural birth

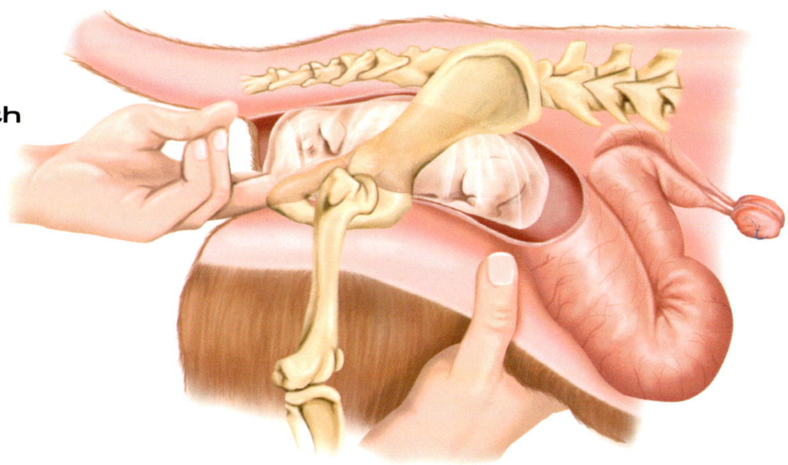

Foetal dystocia

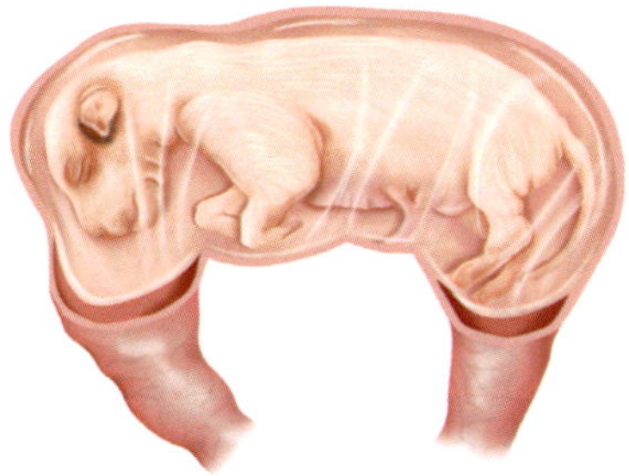
Presentation of the foetus with bent forelegs

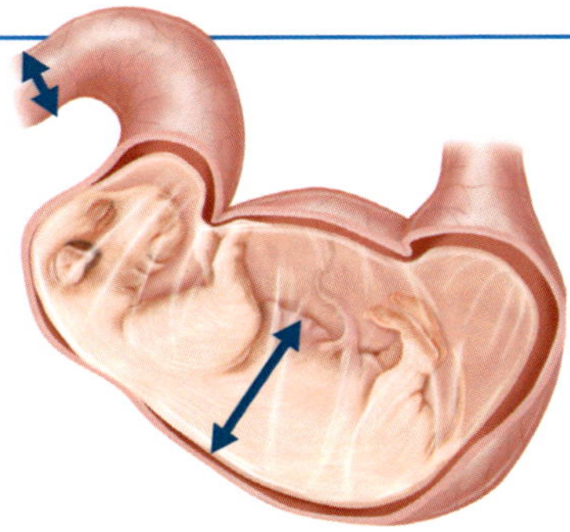
Excessively large foetus

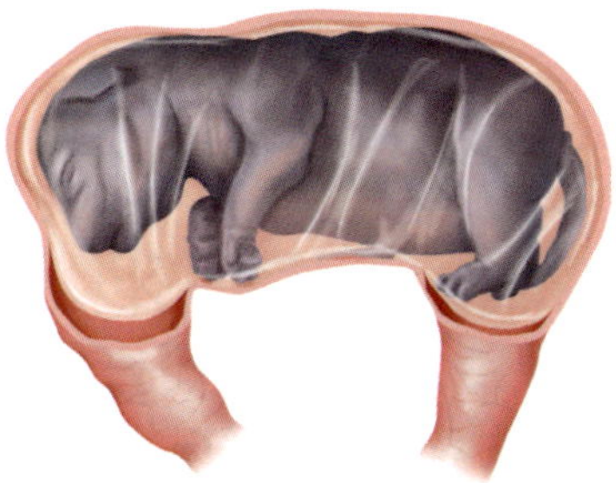
Foetal malformation (anasarca or generalised oedema)

Medical treatment

Calcium gluconate and oxytocin.

Surgical treatment

Caesarean section (necessary in 60-80 % of cases).

UROGENITAL

14 Pyometra

Accumulation of pus within the uterine lumen in not neutered females. It can be opened (vaginal discharge) or closed (no discharge and more severe).

Hormonal therapies for inhibition of oestrus and oestrous cycle disorders are risk factors.

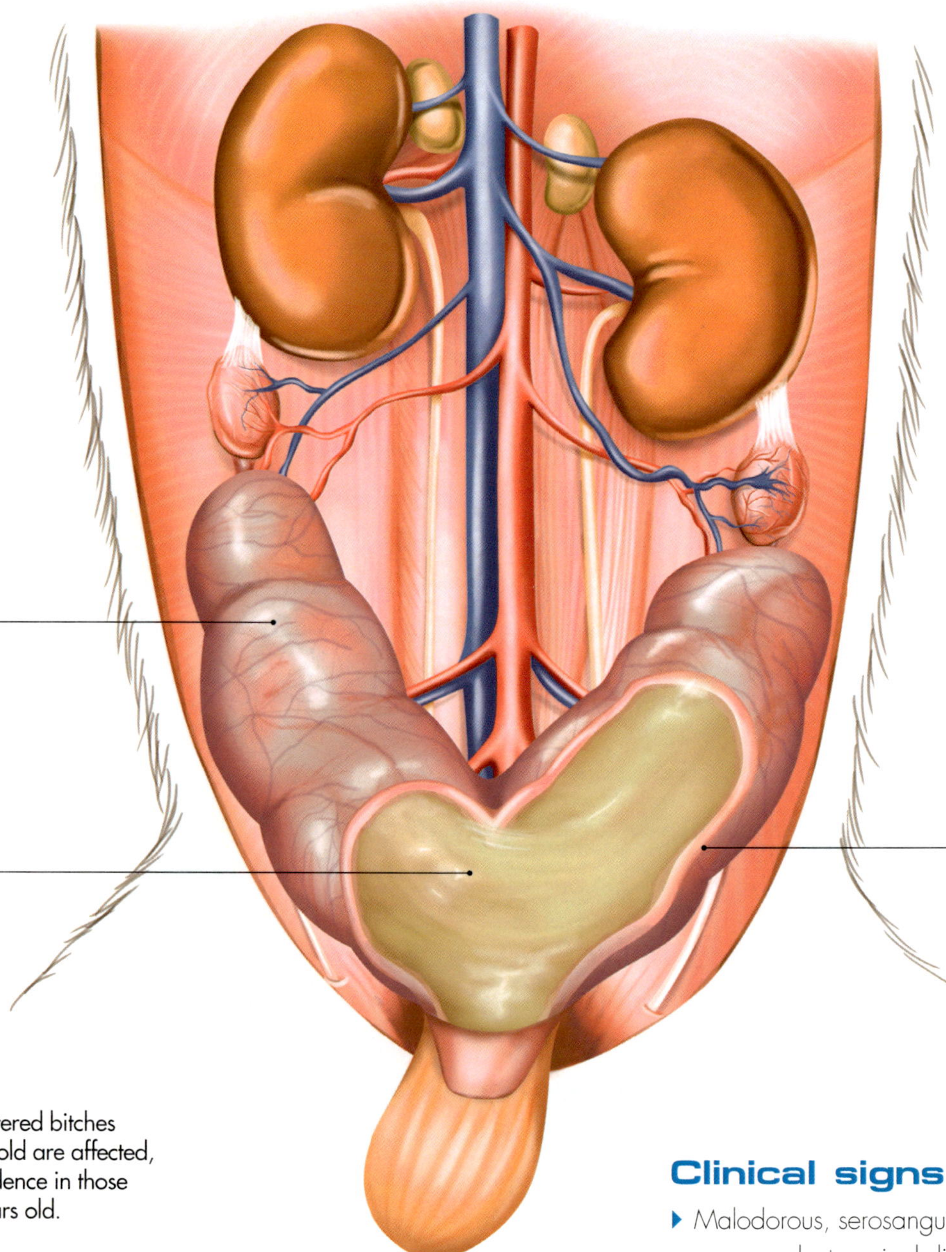

25 % of not neutered bitches under 10 years old are affected, with higher incidence in those older than 4 years old.

Clinical signs

- Malodorous, serosanguineous or mucopurulent vaginal discharge (it will not be observed if it is closed).
- Lethargy, depression, anorexia.
- Polyuria and polydipsia.
- Vomiting, diarrhoea.
- Abdominal distension (closed pyometra).
- There may be fever.

Medical treatment

- Hormonal therapy.
- Fluid therapy.
- Antibiotics.
- Induction of uterine contractions to remove accumulated secretions.

Surgical treatment

Choice: ovariohysterectomy.

UROGENITAL

15 Ovarian diseases

Cysts and neoplasms

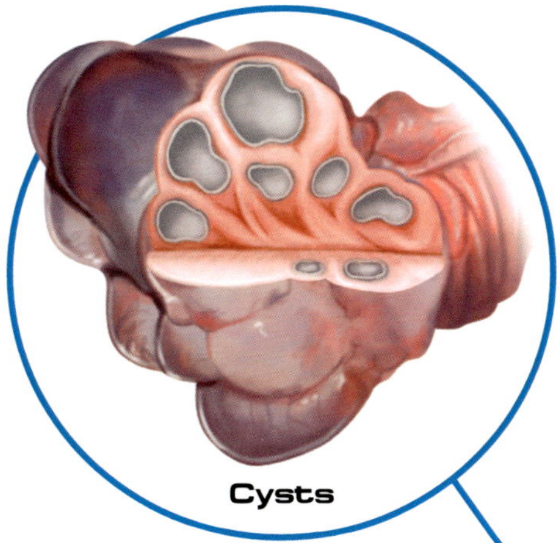

Ovarian cysts

- Liquid-filled lumps with diameters from <1 cm to >10 cm.
- They may be non-functional (epithelial or from ovarian network) and functional, i.e., producing hormones (follicular and luteal).
  - **Follicular cysts:** oestrogen producers. They cause a prolonged proestrus or oestrus, vulvar oedema and bleeding (receptive females).
  - **Luteal cysts:** progesterone producers. They cause a prolonged dioestrus (the bitch not come in heat) and may predispose to cystic endometrial hyperplasia / pyometra.

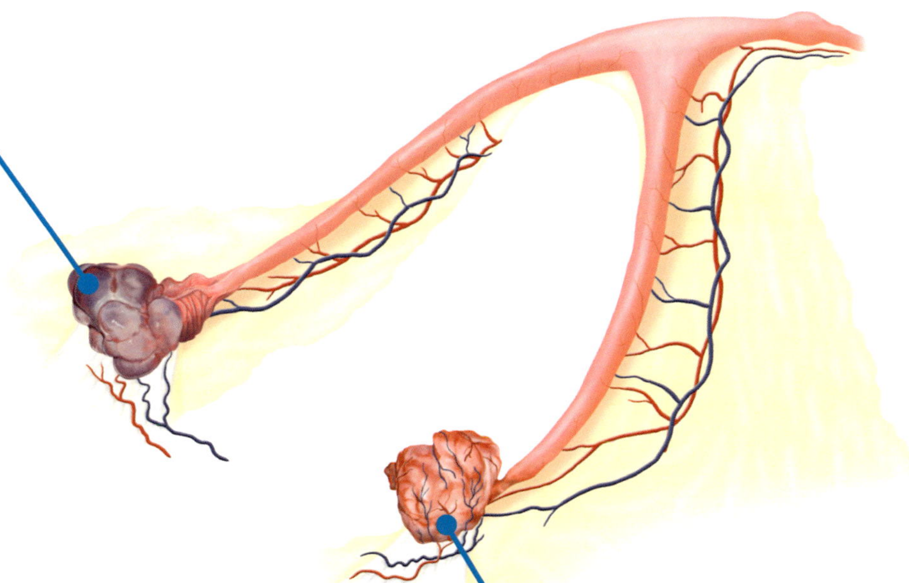

Ovarian neoplasms

Unusual. Several types:

- **Tumours of granulosa cells:** frequent, often oestrogen producers, thus causing changes in the oestrous cycle.
- **Papillary adenoma:** high incidence, benign and usually bilateral. If it grows too much, other organs or healthy ovarian tissue can be pushed.
- **Adenocarcinoma:** the most common malignant ovarian tumour. Vaginal bleeding unrelated to the heat may be produced. Metastasis throughout the abdomen can be produced if it breaks.

Diagnosis is made by hormonal analytics, serial cytology, ultrasound and biopsy.

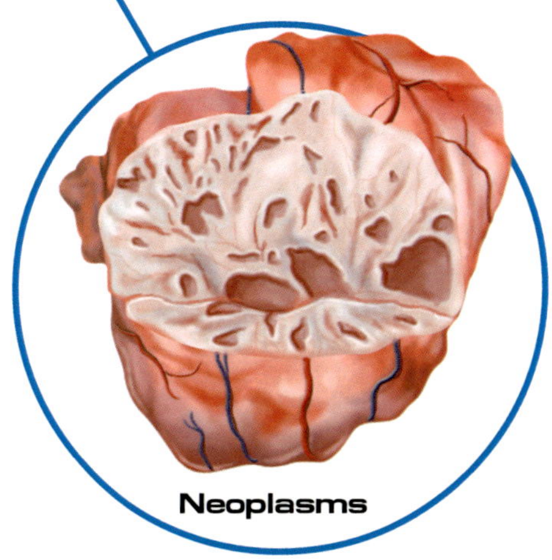

Medical / surgical treatment

For cysts:

- Hormonal treatments for cyst luteinization or luteolysis.
- Choice: ovariohysterectomy.

For neoplasms:

- Ovariohysterectomy immediately.
- The handling of the tumour should be careful to avoid planting of malignant cells in the peritoneum.

UROGENITAL

16 Vaginal hyperplasia and prolapse

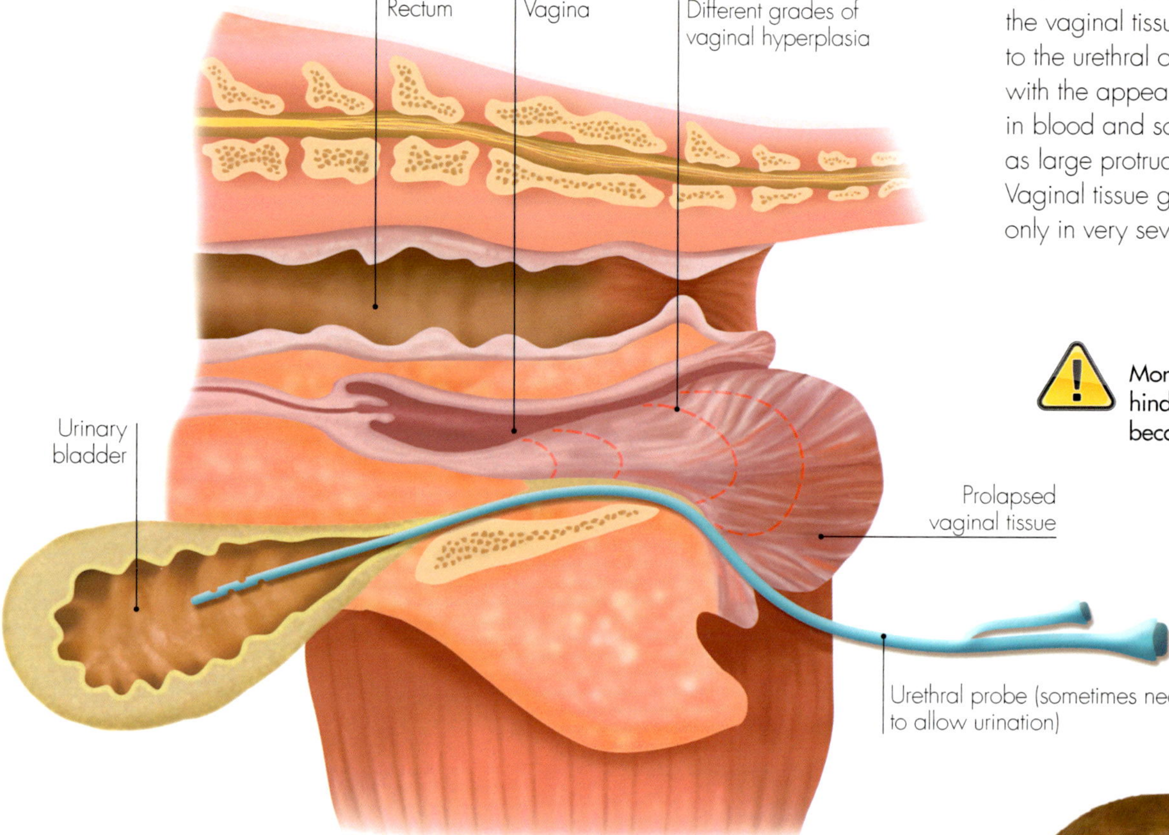

Disease caused by an oedema of the vaginal tissue, frequently cranial to the urethral orifice, which grows with the appearance of oestrogens in blood and sometimes becomes as large protruding from the vagina. Vaginal tissue growth is ring-shaped only in very severe cases.

More severe cases hinder urination, thus becoming urgent.

Do not confuse hyperplasia and vaginal prolapse with uterine prolapse (extremely rare).

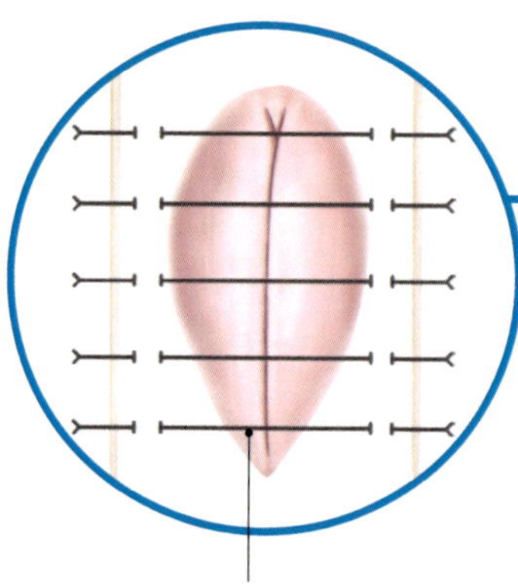

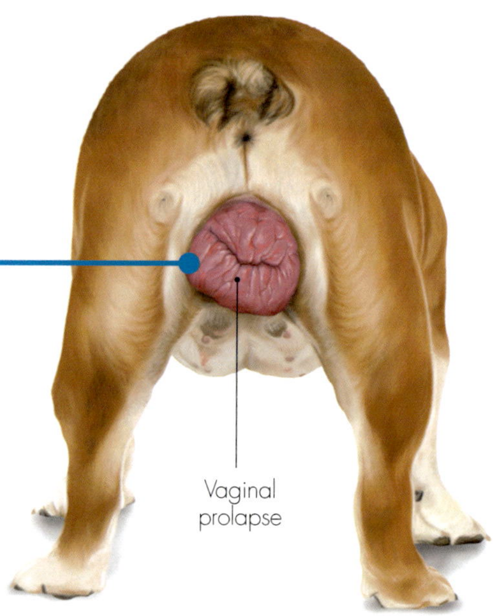

Clinical signs

- Vulvar discharge.
- Painful urination.

Medical / surgical treatment

- Treatment is not necessary in mild cases, being corrected at the end of oestrus.
- Prolapsed vaginal tissue should be kept moist until their size is decreased, either naturally (letting to pass oestrus) or surgically (ovariohysterectomy).
- There are times when the tissue is necrotic and must be surgically removed by episiotomy.
- Applying vulvar retaining sutures may be necessary until hyperplasia is resolved.

UROGENITAL

17 Pseudopregnancy

After dioestrus phase, with progesterone decrease and prolactin increase, the physiological size increase of the mammary glands is frequent. It usually occurs within 6-8 weeks after oestrus (it may vary between 3 to 14 weeks), giving rise a clinical pseudopregnancy which must be treated (only if it occurs exaggeratedly).

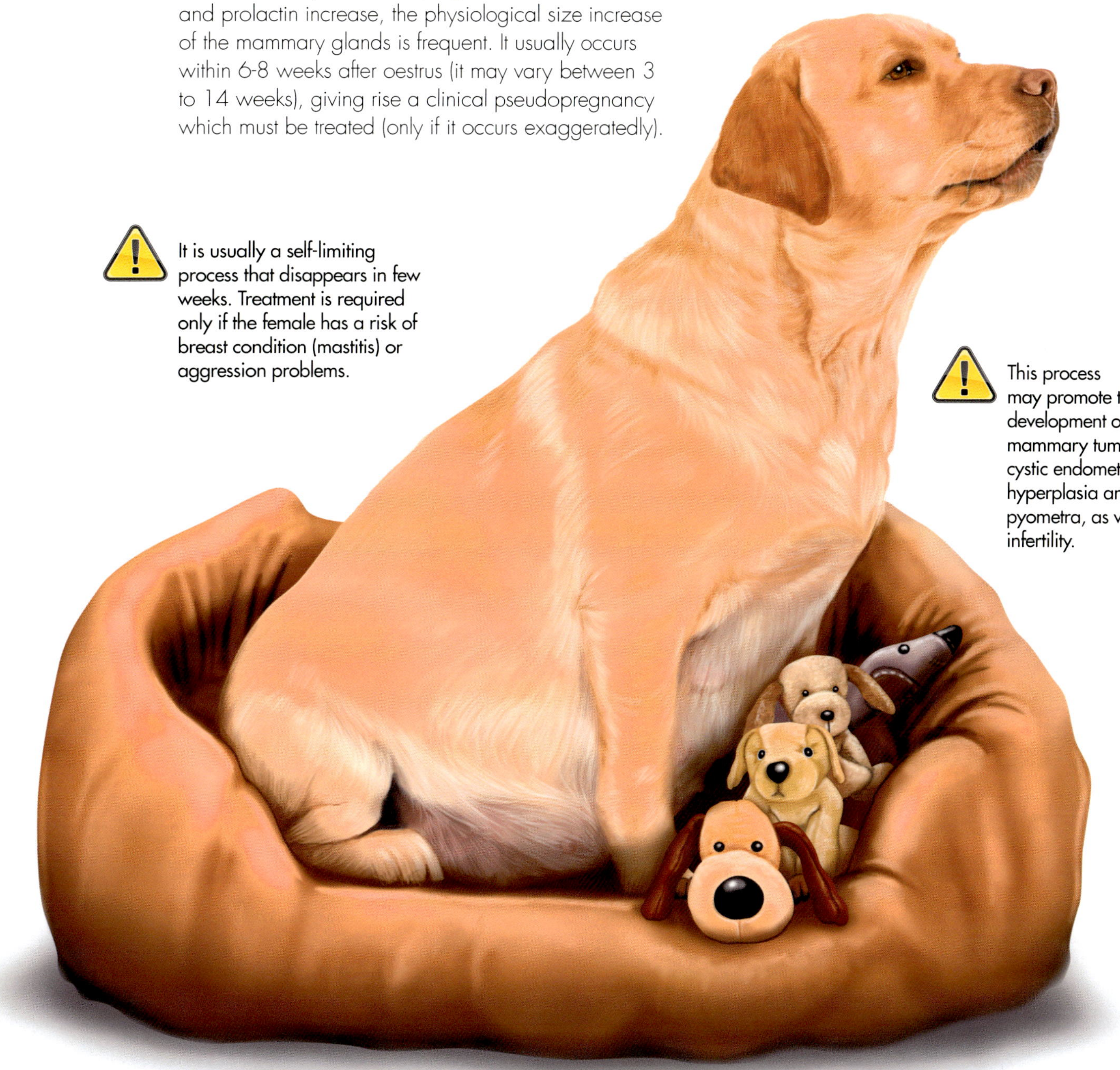

It is usually a self-limiting process that disappears in few weeks. Treatment is required only if the female has a risk of breast condition (mastitis) or aggression problems.

This process may promote the development of mastitis, mammary tumours, cystic endometrial hyperplasia and pyometra, as well as infertility.

Clinical signs

- Swollen mammary gland and abdomen.
- Milk secretion.
- Behavioural changes: nervousness, nesting behaviour, having objects or puppets as puppies.
- Possible maternal aggression.

Medical / surgical treatment

- Antiprolactin drugs may be administered to block the production of prolactin.
- Ovariohysterectomy is the curative treatment in severe and recurrent cases.

UROGENITAL

18 Mammary tumours

The most common tumour in the bitch. 30-50 % of cases are malignant. It may spread to regional lymph nodes and cause metastases mainly in lungs, but also in bone, brain, liver, etc.

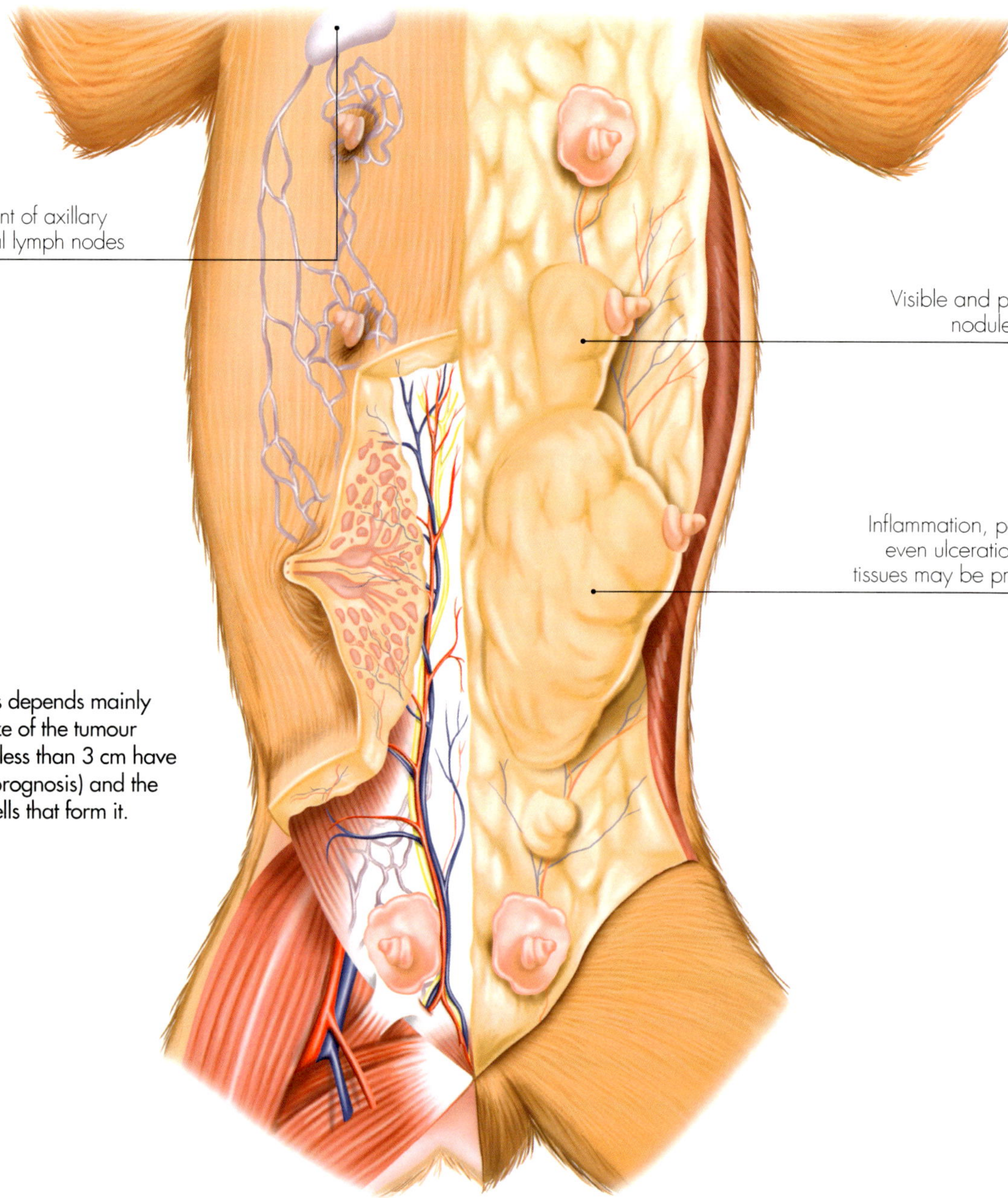

Prognosis depends mainly on the size of the tumour (tumours less than 3 cm have a better prognosis) and the type of cells that form it.

Surgical / medical treatment

- Removal of the affected mammary chain and the regional lymph nodes, with or without chemotherapy and radiotherapy.
- Metronomic chemotherapy is being increasingly used, combining low doses of oral chemotherapeutic agents and COX-2 inhibitors NSAIDs.

65-70 % of canine mammary tumours occur in the 4th and 5th glands.

UROGENITAL

19 Benign prostatic hyperplasia (BPH)

Main process affecting the canine prostate (it occurs in the majority of not neutered older dogs). It is related to an alteration in the androgen / oestrogen ratio, decreasing testosterone and increasing oestrogens with age.

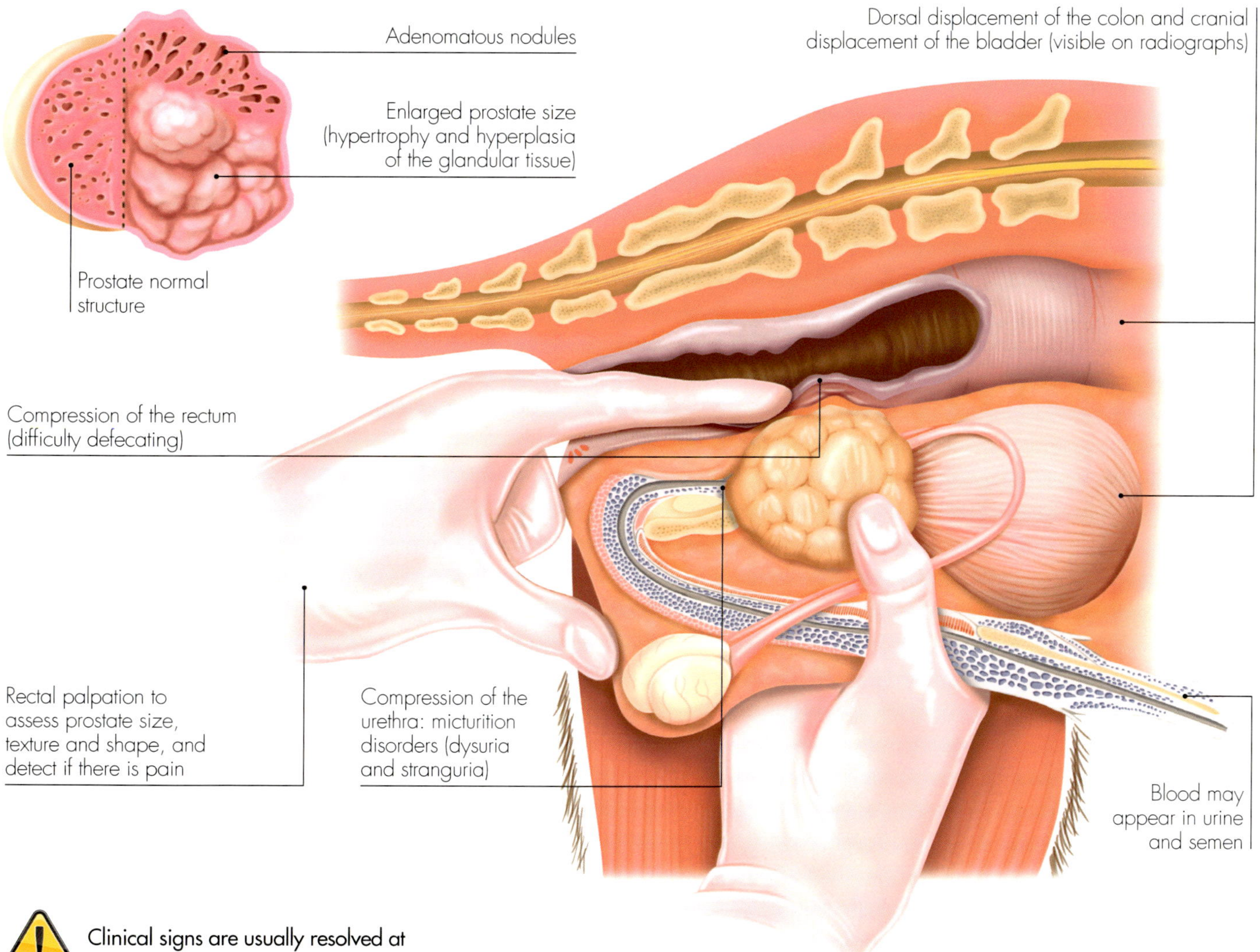

⚠ Clinical signs are usually resolved at 4 weeks after neutering. The prostate size decreases to 70 % at 9 weeks.

Surgical / medical treatment

Treatment should not only be based on surgery (neutering) as good results can be obtained with hormonal treatment.

Paraprostatic cysts

- Usually associated with BPH.
- Formed out of the prostate due to canaliculi obstruction and accumulation of prostatic fluid.
- Treatment includes neutering (essential), ultrasound-guided drainage of the cyst and use of antiandrogens. Besides draining cysts, omentalization technique must be used to avoid relapses.
- Secondary bacterial infections are frequent (prostatic abscess).

UROGENITAL

20 Cryptorchidism

Failure in testicles (one or both) descent into the scrotum, leading to a defect in genital development. Abnormal positions include: intraabdominal, inguinal and subcutaneous.

It is more frequent in purebred dogs (dwarf breeds, Dachshund and Siberian Husky).

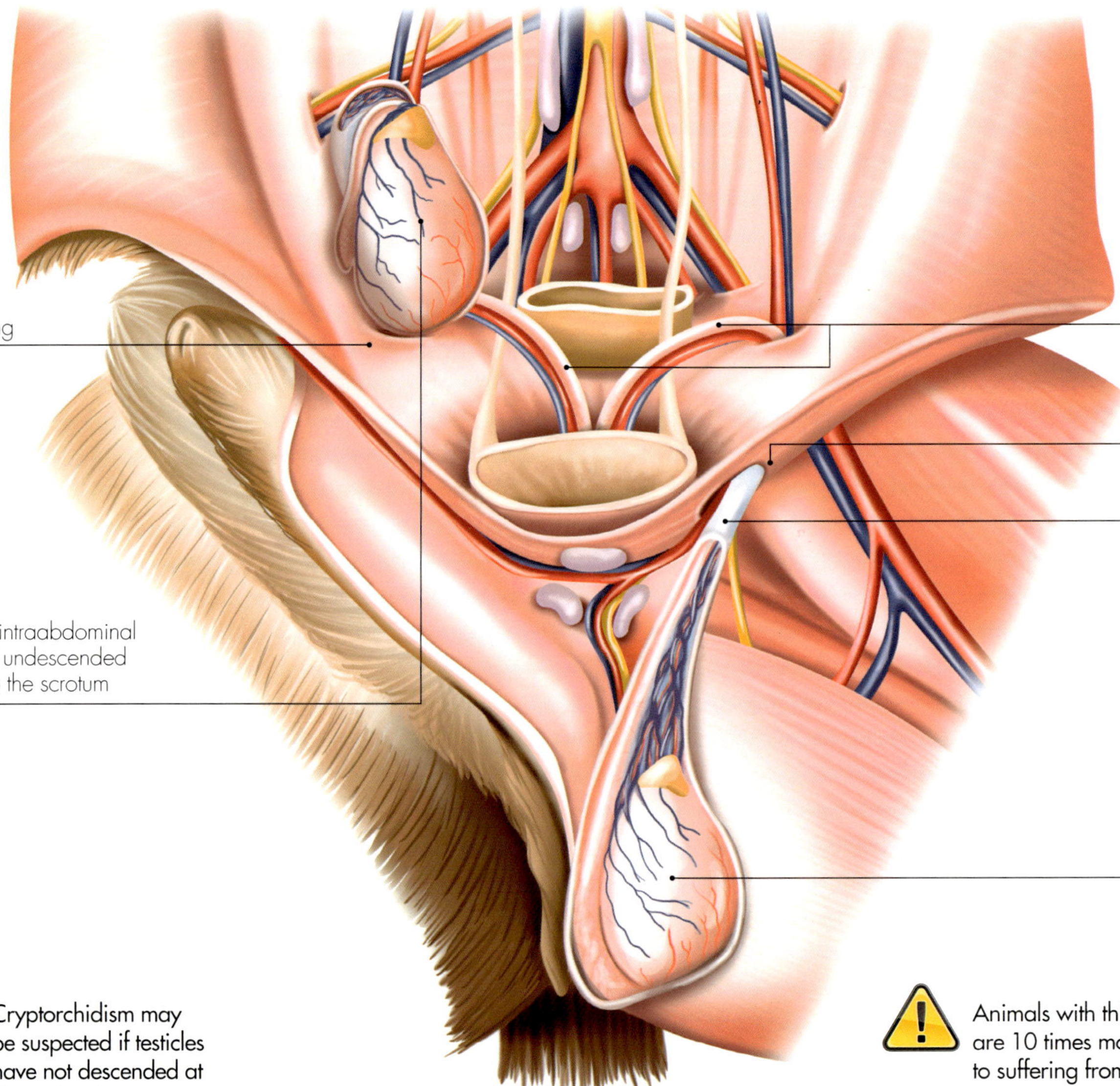

Cryptorchidism may be suspected if testicles have not descended at 2 months of age.

Animals with this condition are 10 times more prone to suffering from testicular tumors, torsion of the spermatic cord, infertility and benign prostatic hyperplasia.

Surgical treatment

Removal of the cryptorchid testicle or preferably both.

Recommendations

A cryptorchid animal should not be used as a stud.
They are fertile, thus they must be controlled, vasectomised or neutered to prevent reproduction.

CARDIORESPIRATORY

21 Brachycephalic syndrome

Surgical treatment

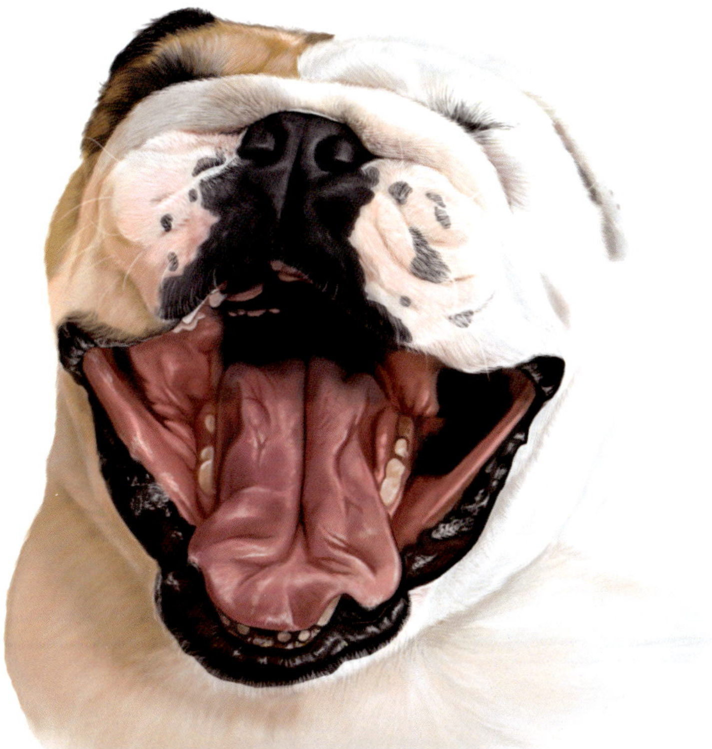

Syndrome which includes several anomalies that make breathing difficult: stenotic nares, elongated soft palate, everted laryngeal saccules, laryngeal collapse, tracheal hypoplasia and thickening of the base of the tongue. The most affected breeds are: English Bulldog, French Bulldog, Boston Terrier, Pekingese, Pug, Shih Tzu, Boxer and Lhasa Apso.

Clinical signs

- Difficulty breathing (dyspnoea).
- Breath sounds (rales and stridor).
- Intolerance to exercise or stress.
- Cyanosis (bluish mucous membranes).
- Possible syncope and collapse.

The most frequent combination is: stenotic nares, elongated soft palate and everted laryngeal saccules (26 % of cases).

Surgical treatment

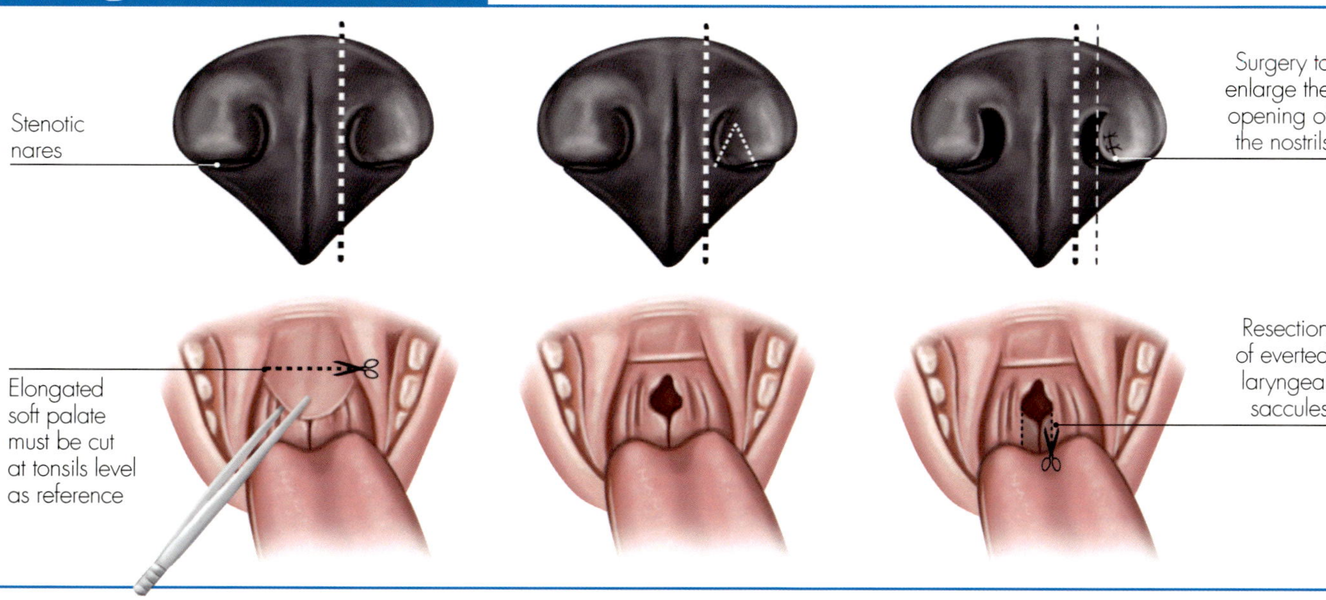

Surgical treatment

- Conventional techniques or laser surgery may be used.
- Correction of stenotic nares.
- Resection of elongated soft palate and everted laryngeal saccules.
- Laryngeal abduction techniques if laryngeal paralysis occurs.

CARDIORESPIRATORY

22 Dilated cardiomyopathy

Normal heart

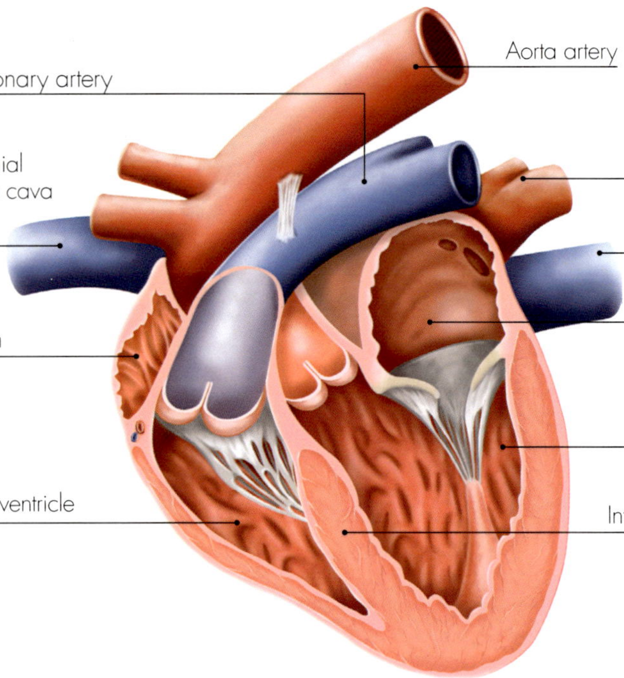

Heart muscle disease usually of unknown origin, typical of large and giant breeds. It also affects Cocker Spaniel. Echocardiography is the diagnostic test of choice.

Clinical signs

- Murmur and gallop rhythm.
- Respiratory difficulty.
- Cardiogenic cough.
- Intolerance to exercise.
- Possible abdominal distension.
- Progressive emaciation and decay.
- Arrhythmias on ECG: sinus tachycardia, atrial fibrillation, ventricular tachyarrhythmias.

Dilated cardiomyopathy

Males are affected 4 times more than females.

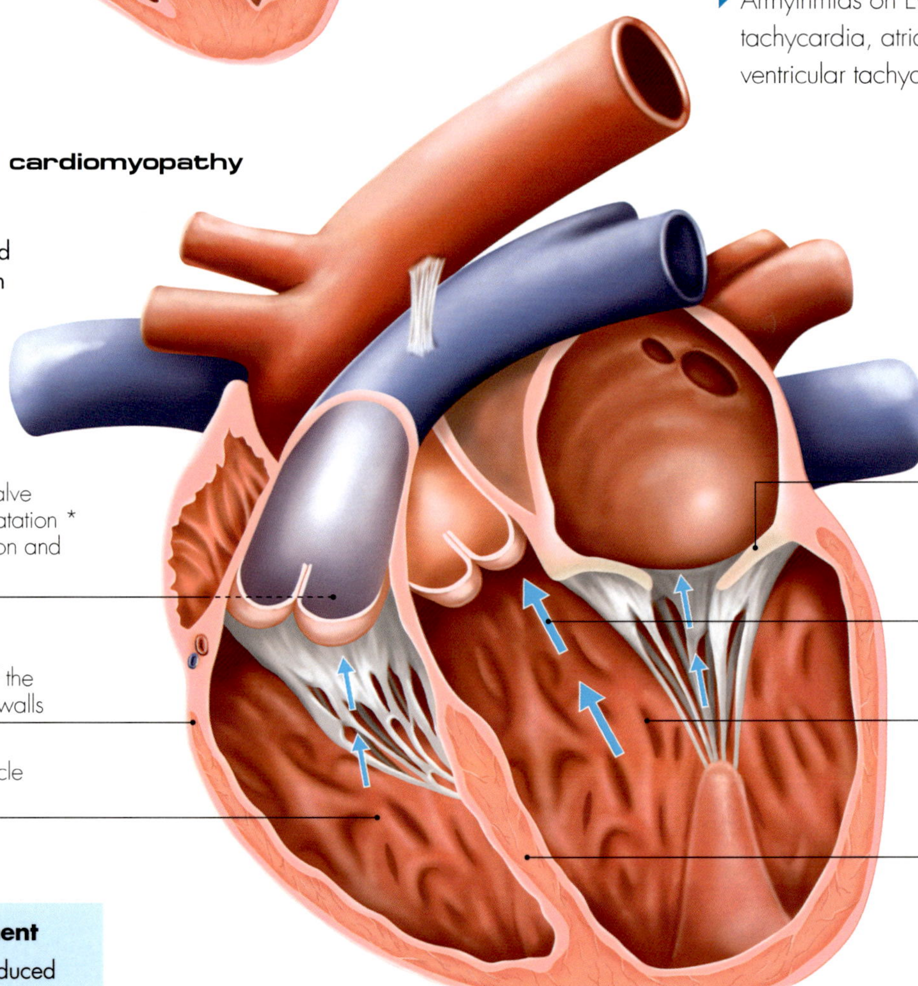

Medical treatment

Drugs, special diet and reduced exercise.

*Is not noticed in the figure because the pulmonary artery is located in a previous level.

CARDIORESPIRATORY

23 Congenital heart diseases

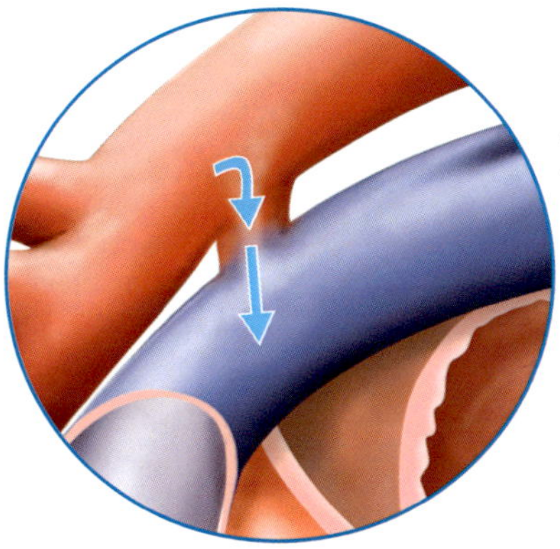

1 PATENT DUCTUS ARTERIOSUS (28 %)

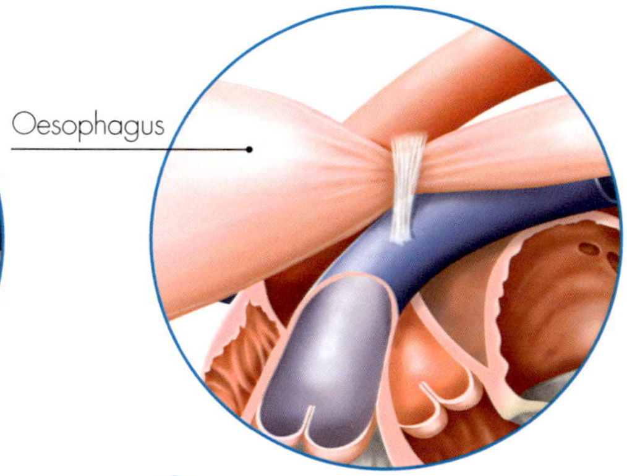

2 PERSISTENCE OF THE RIGHT AORTIC ARCH (8 %)

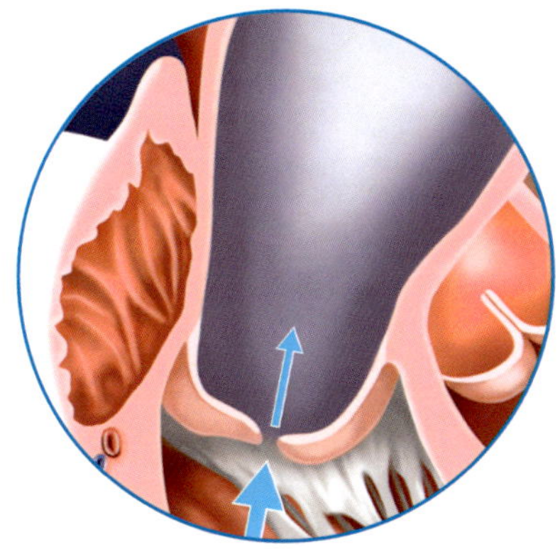

3 PULMONARY STENOSIS (20 %)

Normal heart

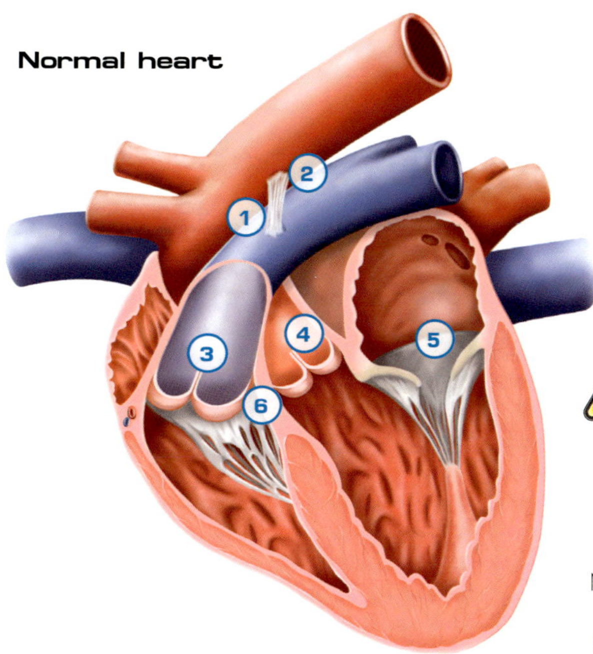

The overall prevalence of congenital heart diseases is 0.8 %.

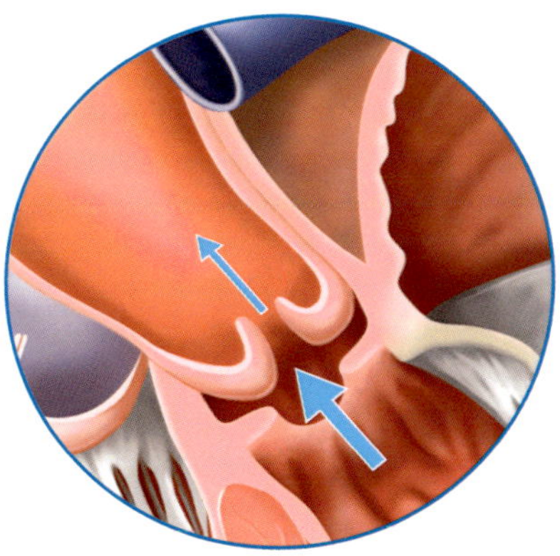

4 AORTIC STENOSIS (14 %)

Diagnosis: combination of clinical signs, radiography, ECG and echocardiography.

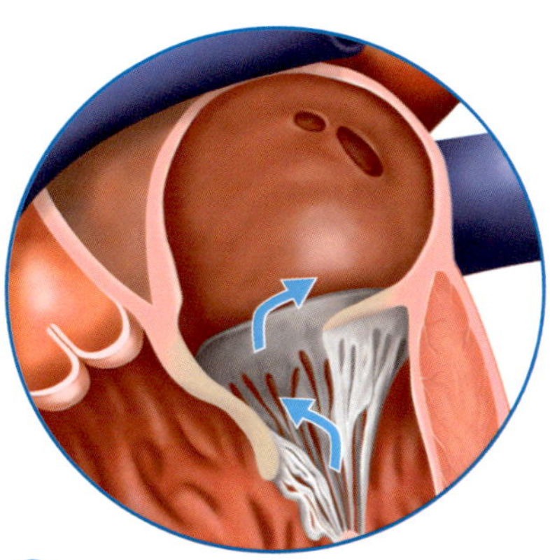

5 MITRAL (MORE FREQUENT) AND TRICUSPID VALVE DYSPLASIA (7 %)

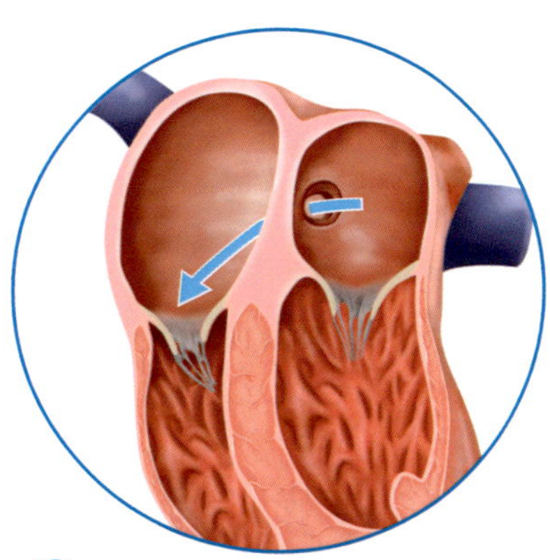

6 INTERATRIAL OR INTERVENTRICULAR SEPTAL DEFECTS (7 %)

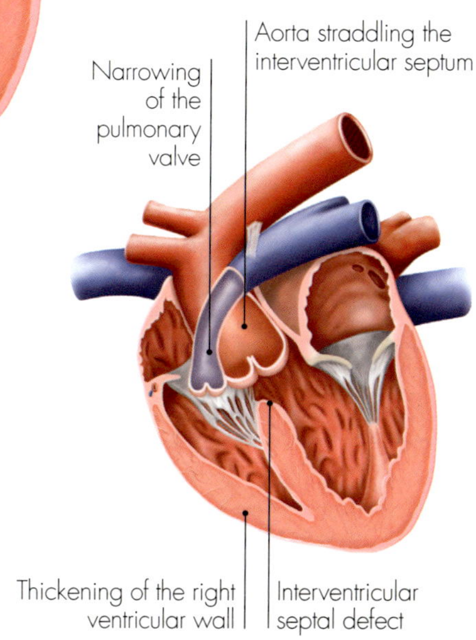

TETRALOGY OF FALLOT (5 %)

CARDIORESPIRATORY

24 Acquired valvular disease

Congestive heart failure (CHF)

The most important cause of heart disease in clinical veterinary, accounting for 75 % of cardiovascular diseases in dogs. Mitral valve is affected in 60 % of cases, while tricuspid valve in 10 %, and 30 % both.

This disease has a chronic and progressive course and leads to CHF.

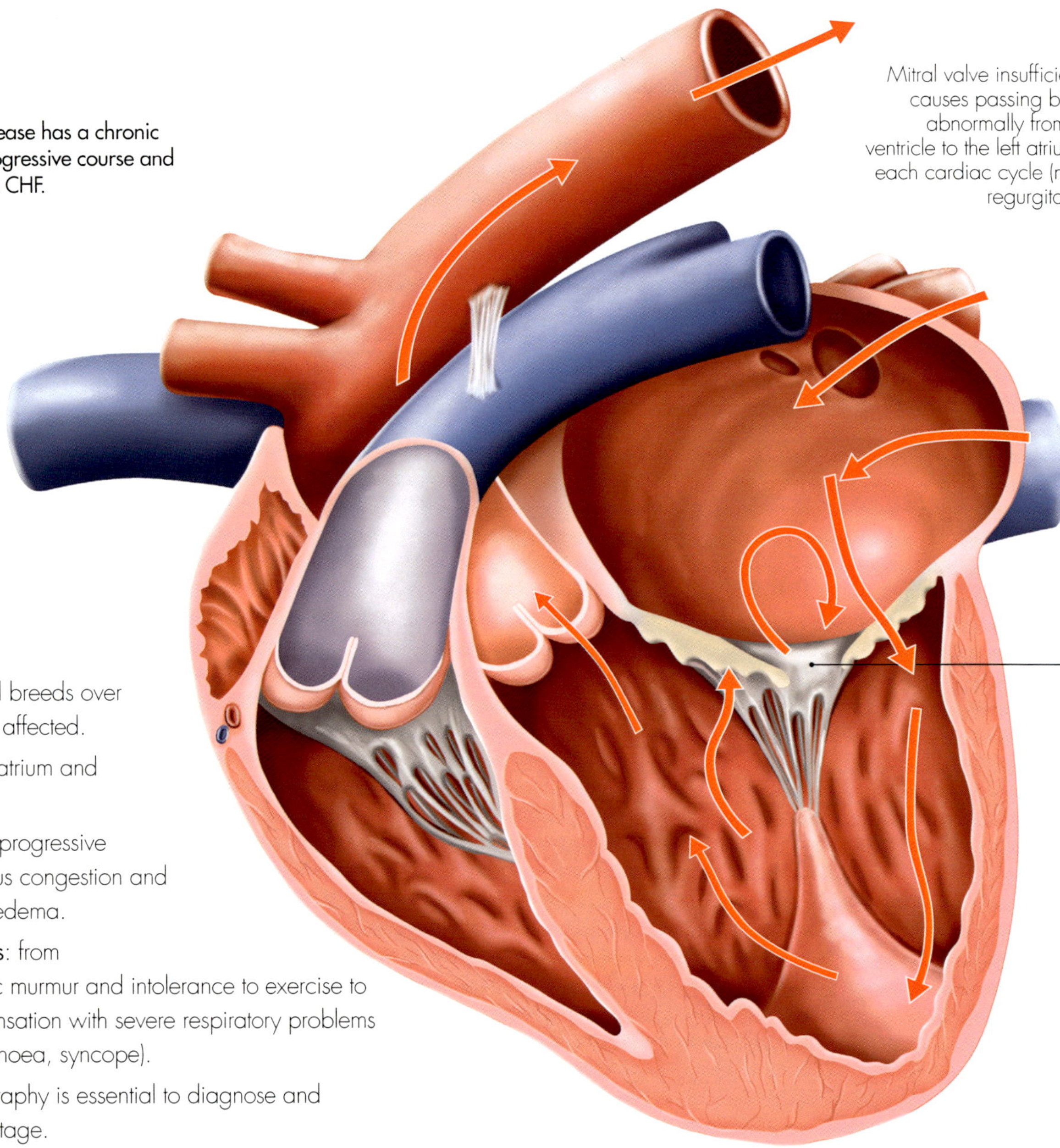

CHF

- 30 % of small breeds over 10 years are affected.
- Enlarged left atrium and ventricle.
- Chronic and progressive course: venous congestion and pulmonary oedema.
- Clinical signs: from asymptomatic murmur and intolerance to exercise to full decompensation with severe respiratory problems (cough, dyspnoea, syncope).
- Echocardiography is essential to diagnose and assess CHF stage.

Medical treatment

Often includes low-sodium diets and drugs of different types (vasodilators, inotropes, antiarrhythmics, diuretics).

There is a genetic form of this disease in Cavalier King Charles Spaniel.

CARDIORESPIRATORY

25 Peritoneal-pericardial-diaphragmatic hernia

The most common congenital pericardial disease in dogs. A permanent communication between the peritoneal and pericardial cavities occurs due to a developmental defect, thus some abdominal organs may surround the heart. The incidence is higher in males (58 %) and there is some breed predisposition in Weimaraner.

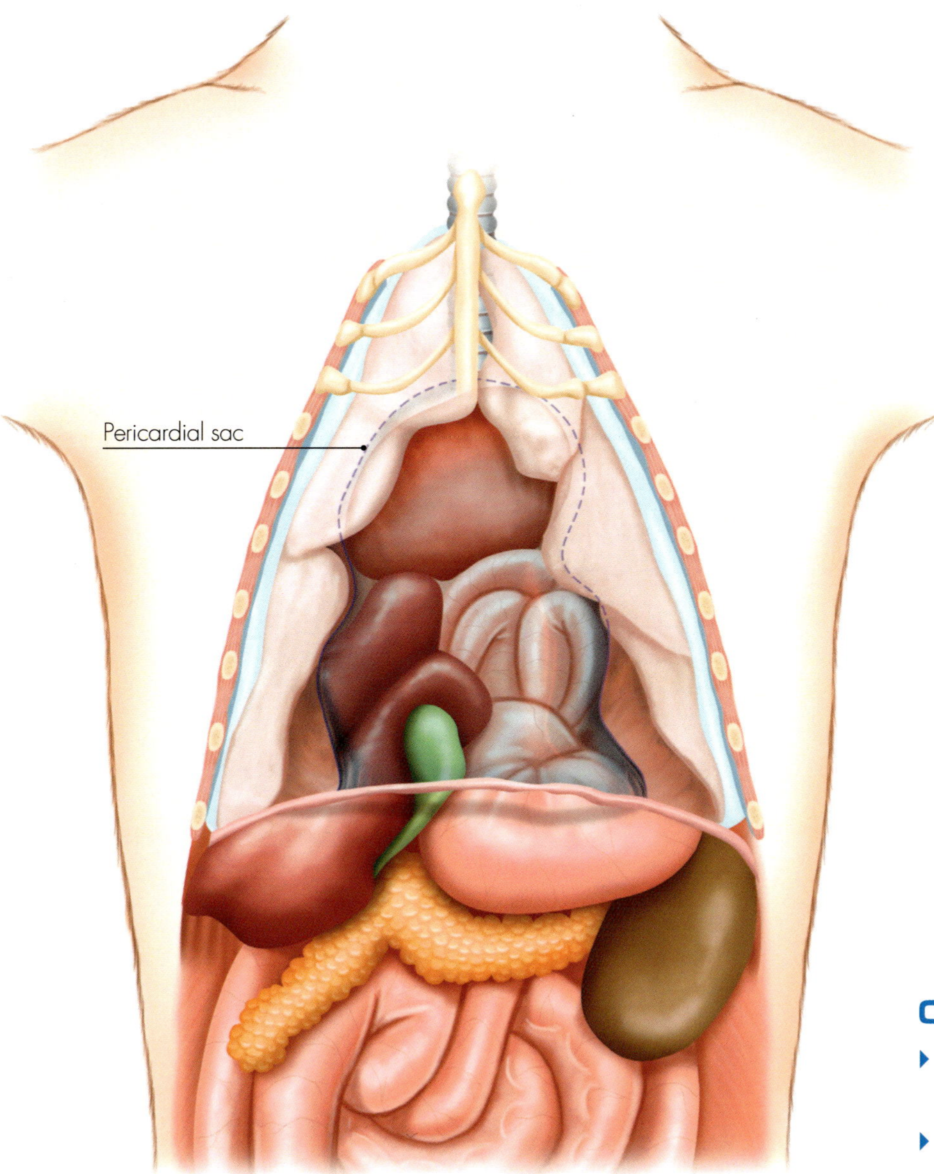

Usually associated with malformations of the sternum, abdominal hernias and heart defects.

Possible associated congenital cardiac abnormalities should be assessed.

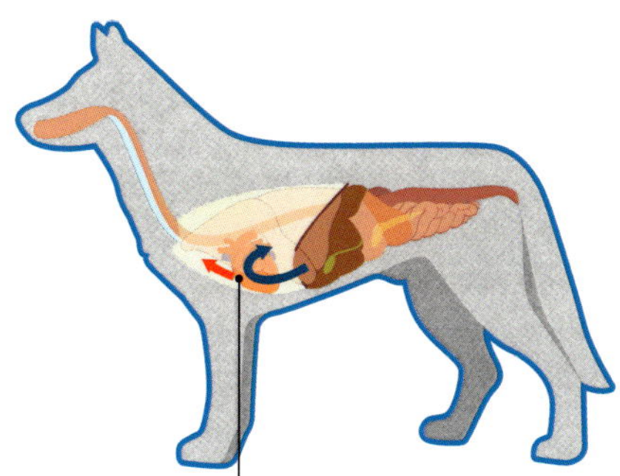

Clinical signs

- Depend on the size of the hernia and the affected organs.
- Gastrointestinal: vomiting, diarrhoea, abdominal pain, anorexia, colic and weight loss.
- Respiratory: dyspnoea, cough, tachypnoea, and intolerance to exercise.
- In some cases the animals are completely asymptomatic.

Surgical treatment

Reduction of the herniated organs and subsequent closure of the defect.

CARDIORESPIRATORY

26 Pneumothorax and pleural effusion

Pneumothorax

Accumulation of air or gas within the pleural space, usually bilateral. Its origin may be spontaneous or traumatic (lung lesion).

Pleural effusion

Accumulation of fluid within the pleural space, which makes breathing progressively difficult.

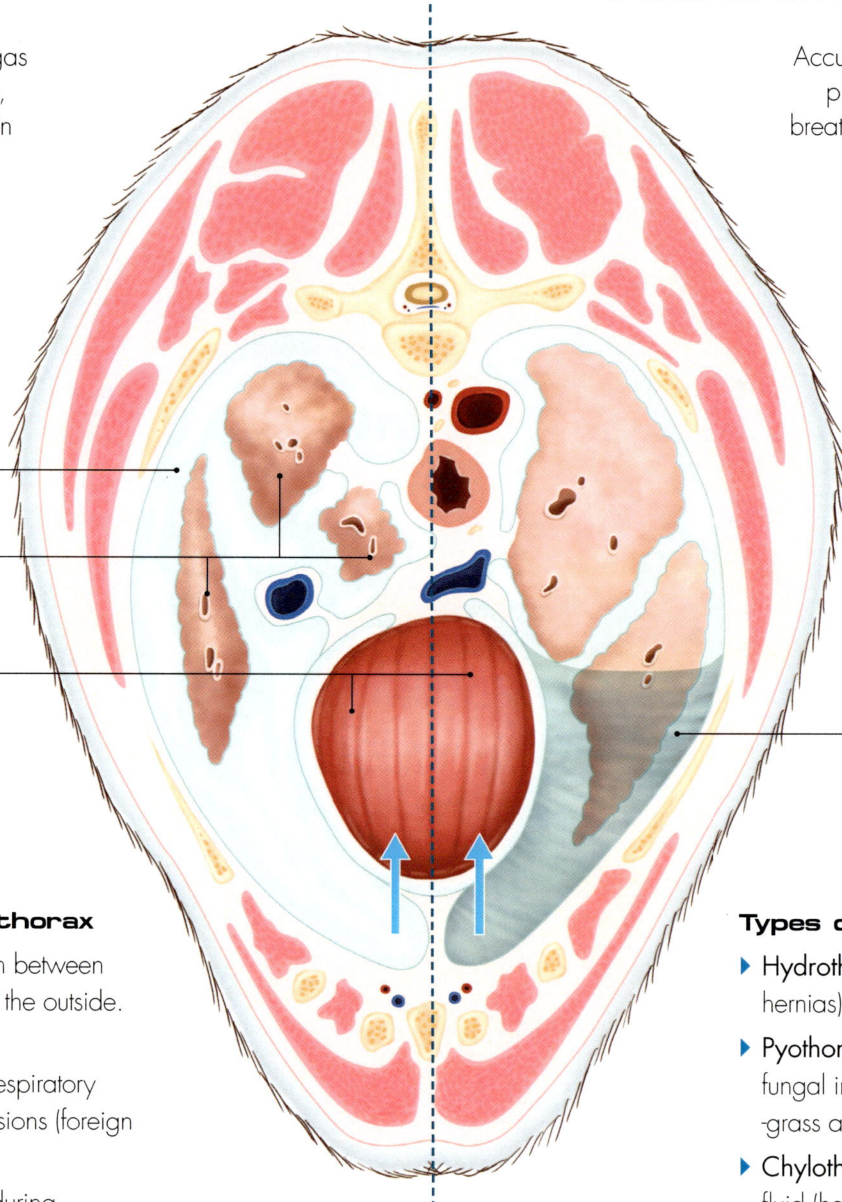

Analysis of pleural fluid obtained by puncture helps to diagnose the cause.

Types of pneumothorax

- **Open:** communication between the pleural space and the outside. Rare in dogs.
- **Closed:** air from the respiratory tree or oesophagus lesions (foreign bodies).
- **Tension:** air entering during the inspiration cannot leave on expiration. It is an emergency and should be corrected quickly.

Types of effusion

- **Hydrothorax:** serous fluid (tumours, hernias).
- **Pyothorax:** pus (bacterial and fungal infections, foreign bodies -grass awns-).
- **Chylothorax:** lymph and chylous fluid (heart disease).
- **Hemothorax:** blood (trauma, coagulopathies, tumours).

Medical treatment

- Thoracic puncture and slow aspiration of the accumulated air or fluid.
- Treatment of the triggering cause of the problem.

Surgical treatment

Placement of a thoracic drainage.

Common clinical signs

- Difficult, shallow and rapid breathing.
- Intolerance to exercise.
- Radiographic (with oxygen therapy): radiopaque lung field, rounded pulmonary edges, loss of cardiac silhouette.

ENDOCRINE

27 Diabetes mellitus in dogs

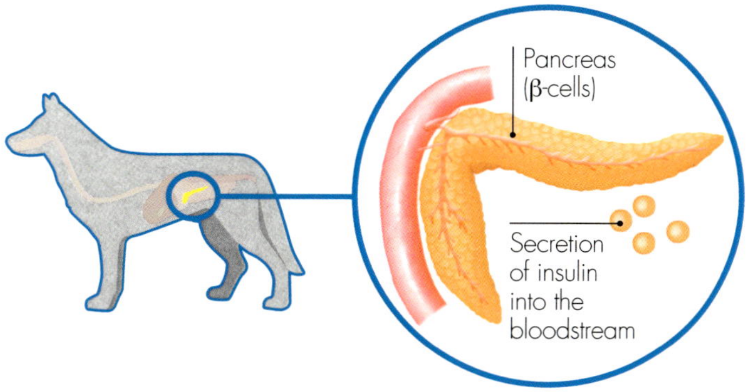

Change in the metabolism of carbohydrates, fats and proteins due to not produce or properly use insulin. The incidence increases in older animals (average: 7-9 years) and females.

Breed predisposition: Poodle, Scottish Terrier, Dachshund, Cairn Terrier and Schnauzer.

Diabetes type 1

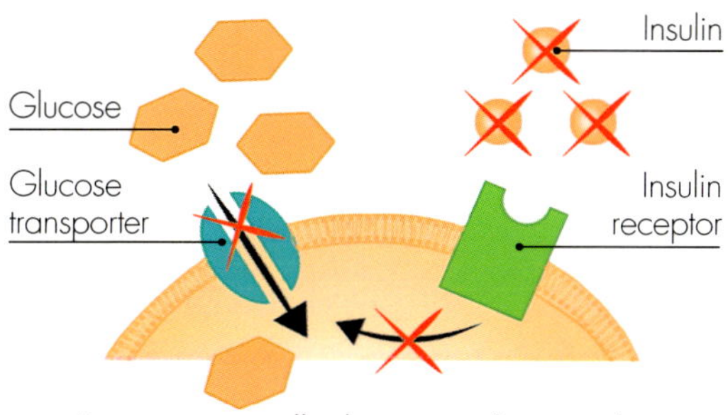

Pancreatic β-cells do not produce insulin

Diabetes type 2

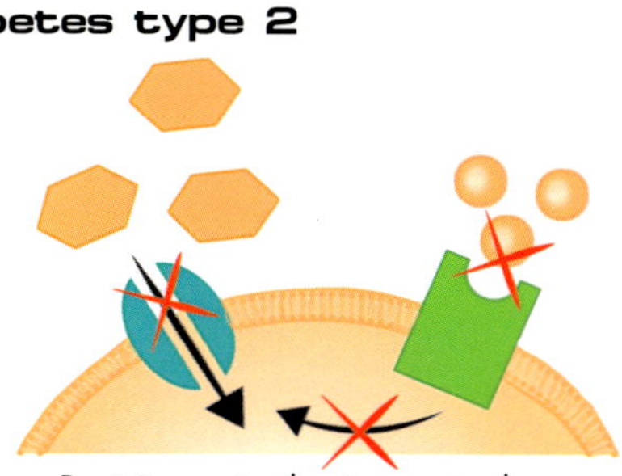

Resistance in the tissues to the action of insulin

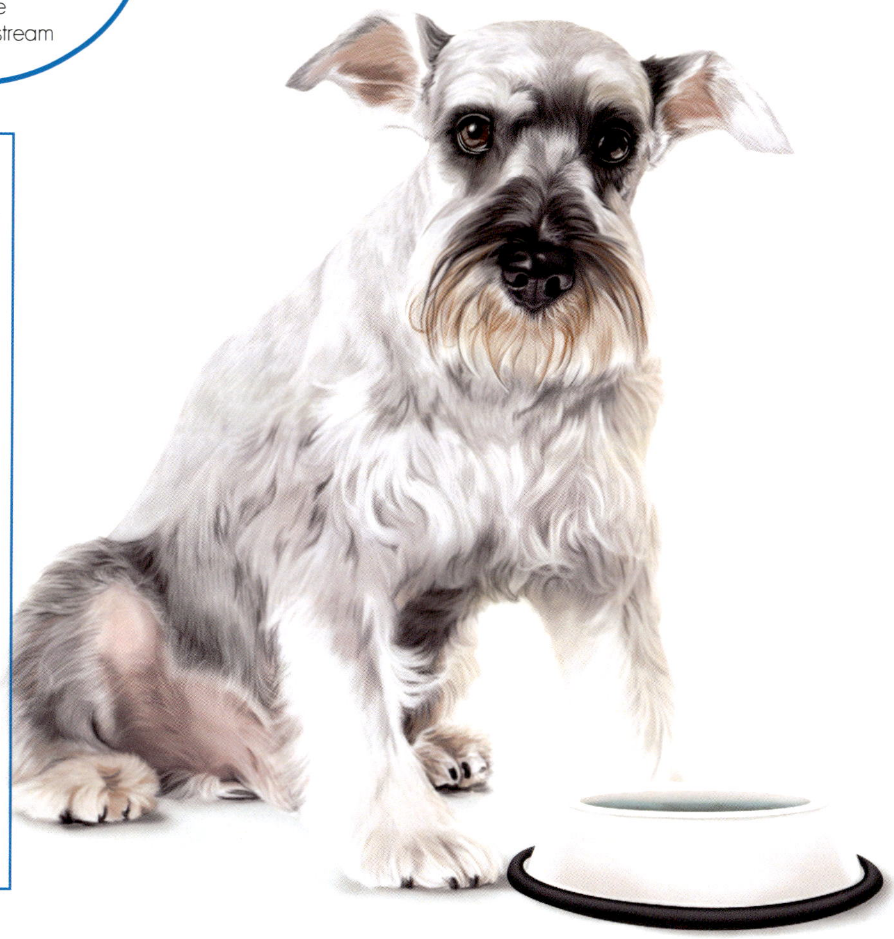

Clinical signs

- Polyuria and polydipsia.
- Polyphagia (increased food intake) and weight loss.
- Persistent presence of glucose in blood and urine.

Diabetes causes chronic complications such as blindness from cataract formation, chronic pancreatitis and recurrent urinary tract, respiratory system and skin infections, as well as diabetic ketoacidosis (hypovolaemic shock associated with severe electrolyte abnormalities and multiorgan failure).

Medical treatment

- Insulin.
- Treatment of triggering factors.
- Monitor treatment through regular analyses (glucose curves, glycosuria).

Dietary treatment

Diet low in carbohydrates and high in protein.

Recommendations

- Regular exercise prevents hyperglycaemia and improves insulin absorption.
- Females neutering: the best control of diabetes.

ENDOCRINE

28 Hyperadrenocorticism

Cushing's syndrome

Persistent and chronic elevation of plasma concentrations of glucocorticoids. It may be endogenous (disturbance of the pituitary or adrenal glands) or exogenous (repeated administration of glucocorticoids).

The most common age of onset is 8-12 years, with a higher incidence in females.

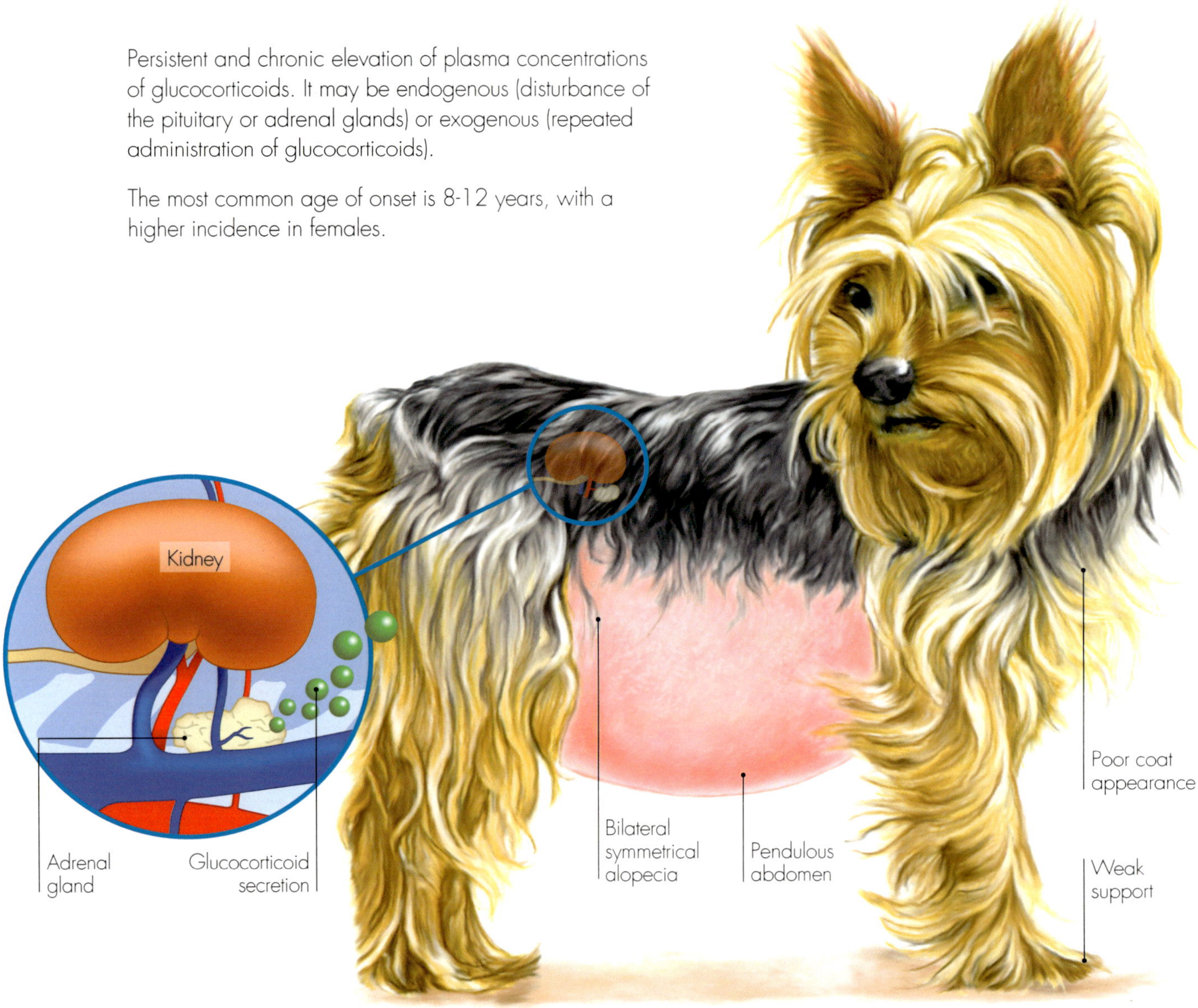

Breed predisposition, especially Poodle and Dachshund, but also Beagle, Boston Terrier and Boxer.

Clinical signs

- Polyuria and polydipsia.
- Polyphagia.
- Enlarged abdomen, hepatomegaly.
- Bilateral symmetrical alopecia, very thin skin, pyoderma.
- Panting, muscular weakness in supporting and lethargy.

Medical treatment

- The underlying cause of hyperthyroidism.
- Administration of inhibitors of the adrenal gland.

Surgical treatment

In case of tumours of the adrenal glands (adrenalectomy).

ENDOCRINE

29 Hypoadrenocorticisim

Addison's disease

Deficit in the production of glucocorticoids, mineralocorticoids or both by the adrenal glands. It can be primary or secondary. The incidence is higher in young and middle-aged adults, and intact females.

Primary hypoadrenocorticism

Involvement of the adrenal glands:

- ↓ Glucocorticoids (cortisol).
- ↓ Mineralocorticoids (aldosterone).

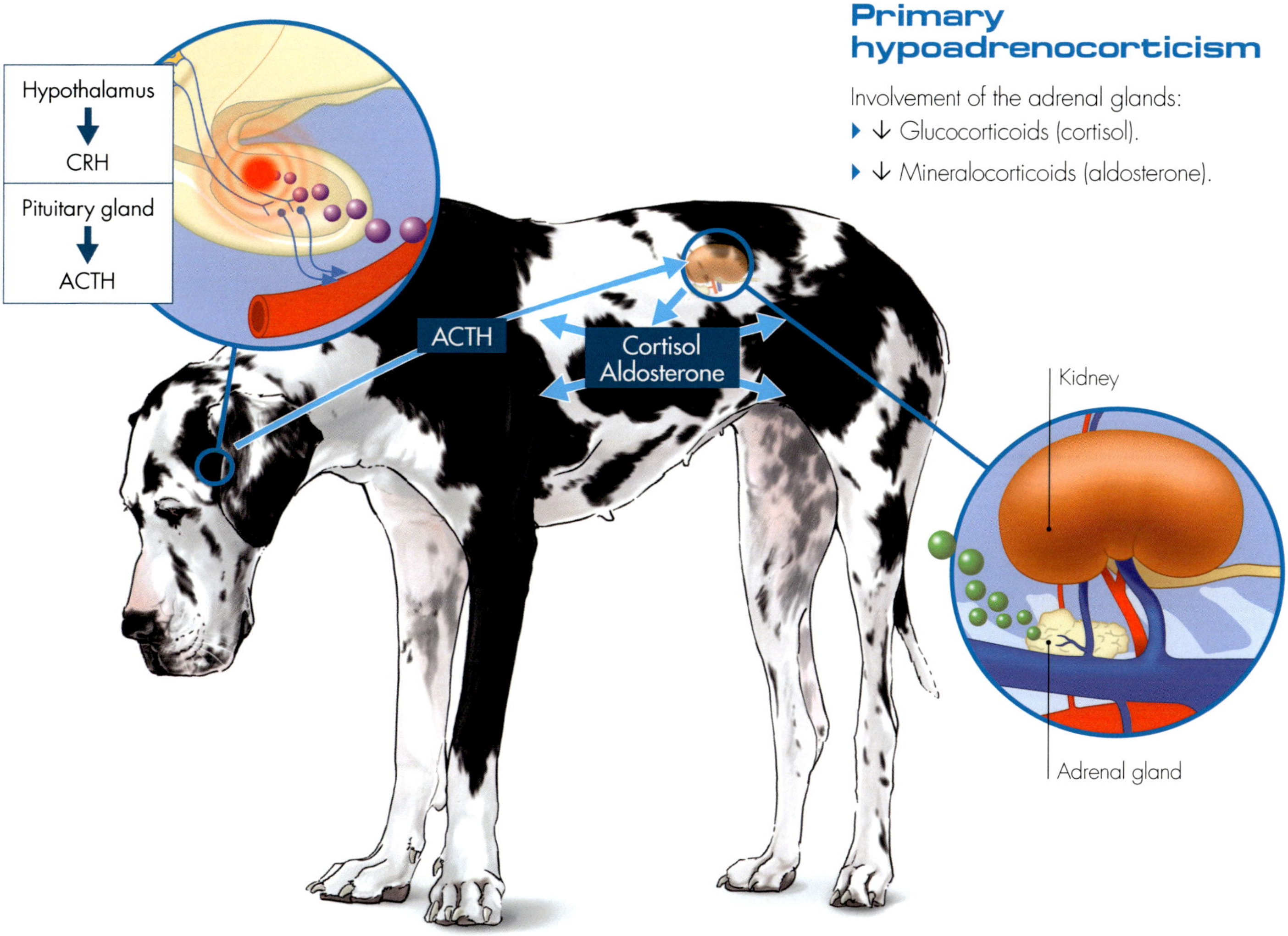

Secondary hypoadrenocorticism

- Involvement of the hypothalamus or pituitary gland (alterations in CRH and ACTH secretion).
- Exogenous glucocorticoid administration.

Clinical signs

- Acute progression: collapse to stress. Besides, weak pulse, bradycardia, abdominal pain, vomiting, diarrhoea, dehydration and hypothermia.
- Chronic progression (more frequent): nonspecific signs and exacerbated by stress, such as anorexia, vomiting, lethargy, depression and weakness.

Medical treatment

Mineralocorticoid and / or glucocorticoid supplementation.

Recommendations

Important: reducing treatments gradually with corticosteroids.

ENDOCRINE

30 Hypothyroidism in dogs

Deficiency in the secretion of thyroid hormones by the thyroid gland. Both young (congenital or acquired) and adults are affected. It may be primary, secondary or tertiary.

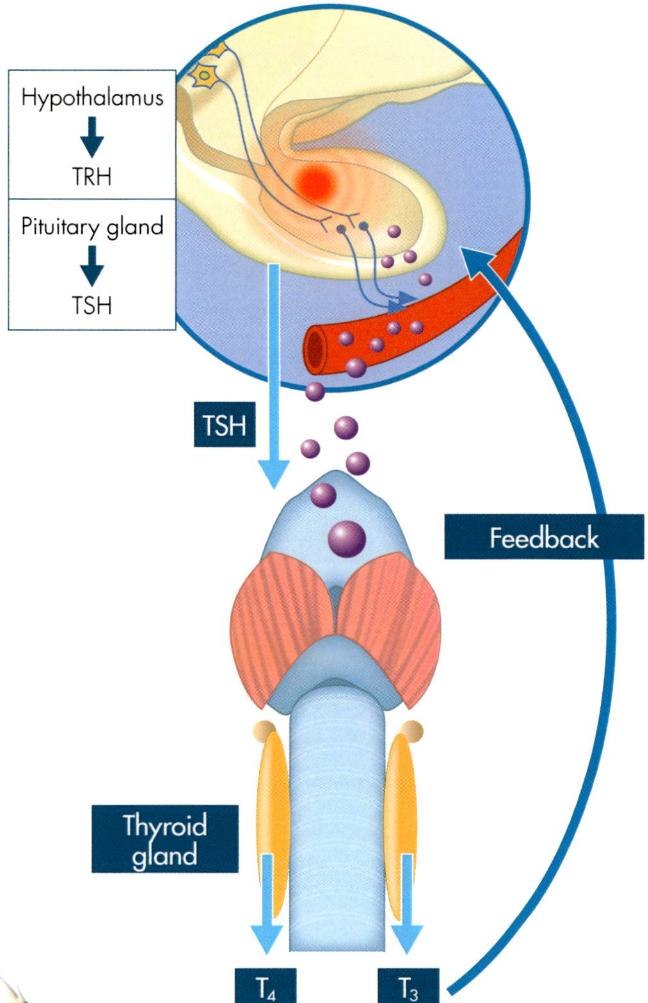

Primary hypothyroidism (>95 %)

Involvement of the thyroid gland (↓ T4 and T3), usually by an autoimmune process (autoimmune thyroiditis).

Secondary or tertiary hypothyroidism (<5 %)

Involvement of the pituitary gland or hypothalamus (alteration in TSH and TRH secretion).

Dogs of medium or large size are affected, especially Golden Retriever, Irish Setter, Doberman, Beagle, Cocker Spaniel, Dachshund, Miniature Schnauzer and Airedale Terrier.

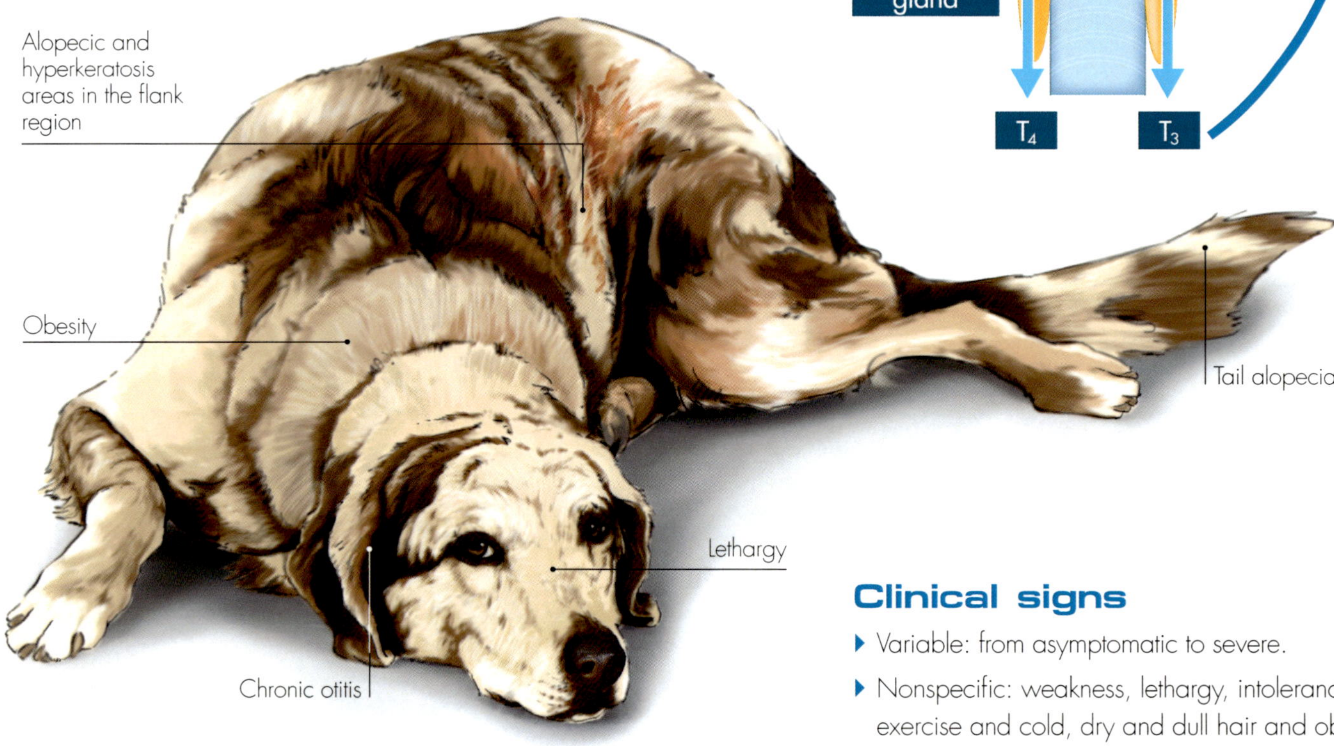

Medical treatment

Lifetime supplementation with thyroid hormones.

Clinical signs

- Variable: from asymptomatic to severe.
- Nonspecific: weakness, lethargy, intolerance to exercise and cold, dry and dull hair and obesity.
- By systems: skin (symmetrical alopecia, thickened skin, infections), neuromuscular, cardiac, reproductive, ocular, behavioural disorders, etc.

SKIN AND ADNEXA

31 Skin structures in dogs

Skin layers

1. Epidermis.
2. Dermis.
3. Subcutaneous tissues or hypodermis.

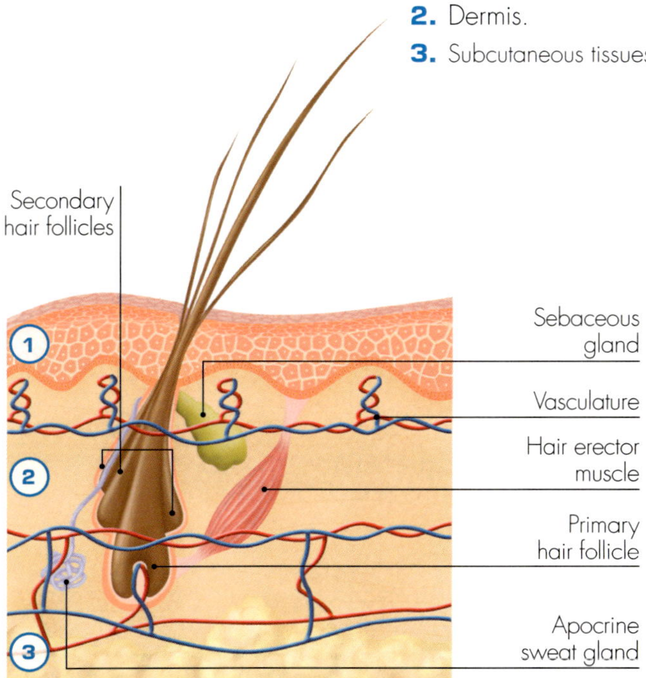

NORMAL HAIR

Hair moulting occurs twice a year (spring and the onset of winter). In dogs living inside the house, where there are no major changes in temperature, moulting can continue throughout the year.

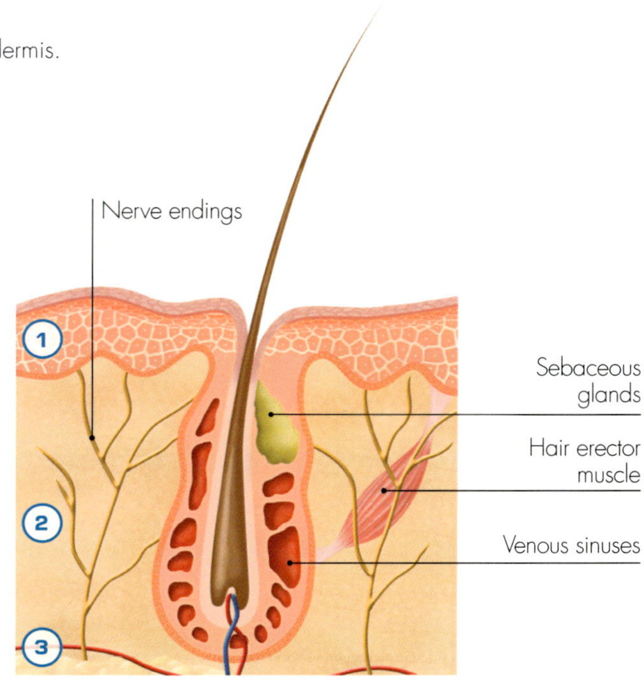

TACTILE HAIR OR VIBRISSA

Although not as sensitive to changes in pressure and air currents as in cats, dogs also have these specialised hairs in different areas of the face.

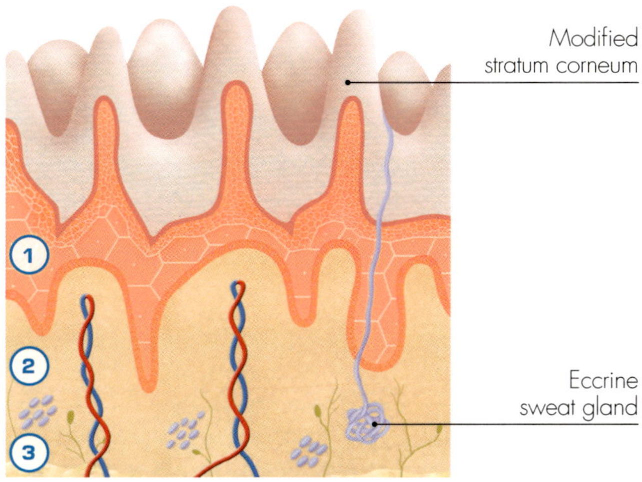

PAW PAD

- Highly modified skin areas consisting of adipose cells, which cannot be compressed, and elastic areas.
- Their sweat glands are involved in the marking of territory.

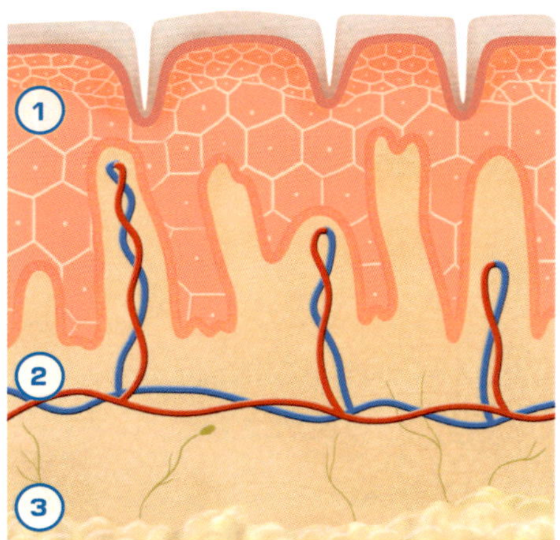

NASAL EPITHELIUM (muzzle)

- The moisture and temperature of the dog's nose are not always indicative of his health; it may be hot and dry by previous sun exposure.
- If it is not pigmented, it is better protecting it from sunlight.

SKIN AND ADNEXA

32 Ectoparasites

Fleas and ticks

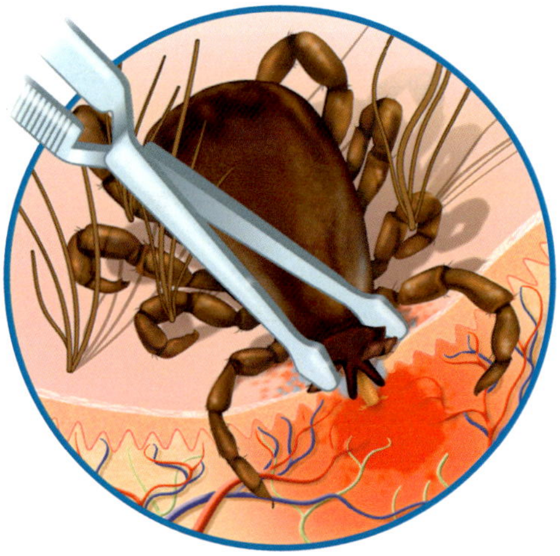

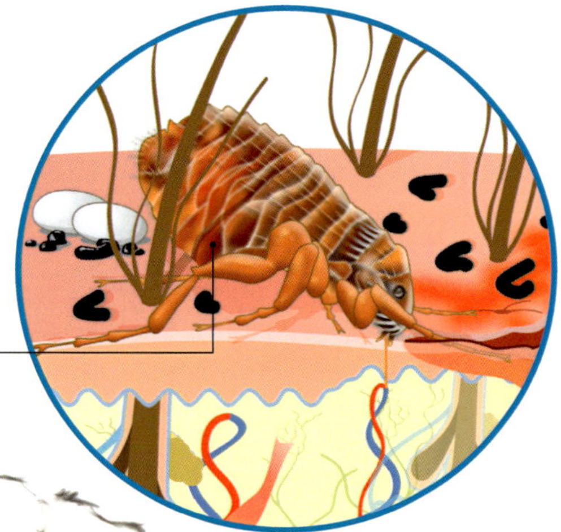

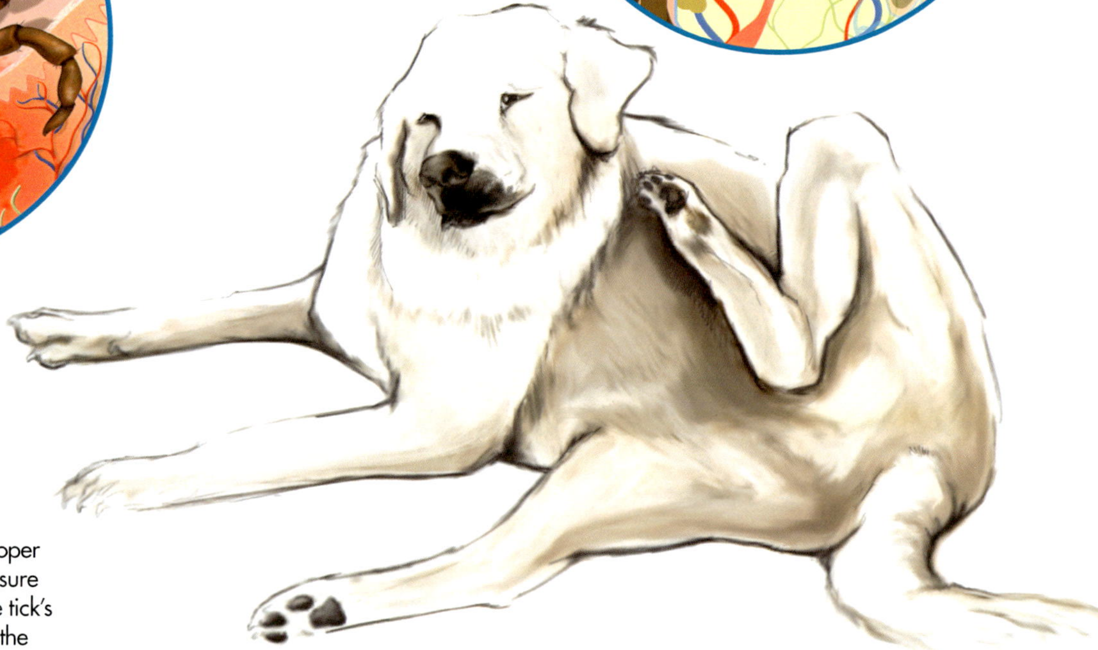

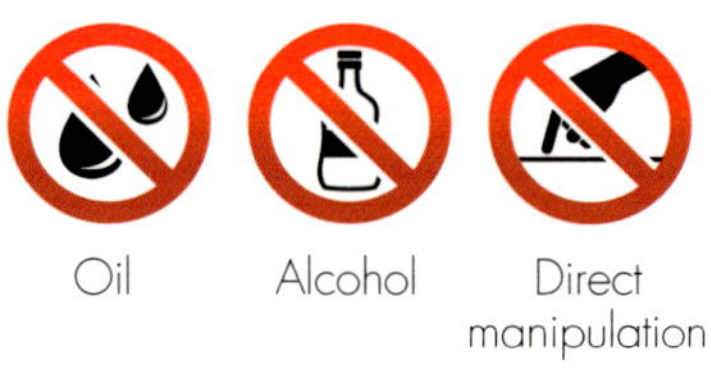

It is important to follow a proper tick removal technique to ensure there are no remnants of the tick's feeding apparatus and that the possible pathogenic agents cannot be eliminated in the bloodstream.

Fleas can be detected by means of a fine-tooth comb or by looking for their faeces in the dog's hair.

Tick infestation

- They are usually of the genus *Rhipicephalus*.
- They are mainly located in areas of difficult access for the animal: eyelids, back and lower back, ears, etc.
- They may transmit infectious diseases (ehrlichiosis, Lyme's disease, babesiosis, etc.).
- **Clinical signs:** redness and mild itching, scabs and small nodules at the sites of attachment, otitis externa in case of a large number of parasites and even paralysis.

Medical treatment

- Application of anti-tick products on the dog and on the environment.
- Thorough cleaning of the environment in the case of fleas (they lay 40 eggs/day on average in the host environment).
- Symptomatic treatment of hypersensitivity.

Hypersensitivity to flea bites

- Frequent condition caused by an allergic reaction to their saliva.
- Fleas can transmit infectious diseases (rickettsiosis, bartollenosis, haemoplasmosis) and parasitic diseases (tapeworm infection).
- Greater predisposition in atopic dogs.
- **Clinical signs:** variable pruritus, alopecia, erythema, papules, scabs, excoriation, hyperpigmentation and lichenification.
- Location of the lesions: caudal part of the back, flanks, tail and perineum.

SKIN AND ADNEXA

33 Types of mange

Disease transmissible to humans (zoonosis).

Sarcoptic mange

Caused by the mite *Sarcoptes scabiei*. It digs skin furrows or galleries, where the female lays eggs. It produces severe pruritus and allergic reactions.

Clinical signs

- Severe pruritus.
- Scaly papules and scabs.
- Excoriations and alopecia.

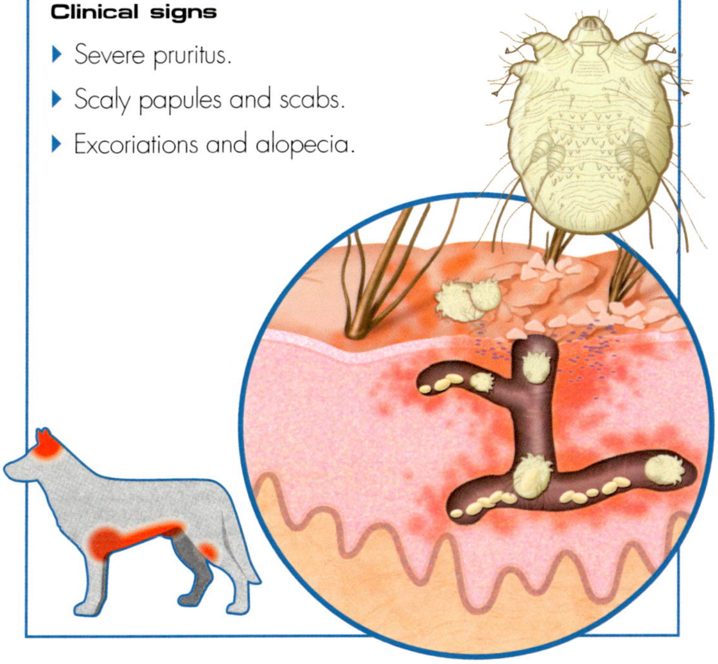

Demodectic mange

Caused by the mite *Demodex canis* (inside the hair follicles). It is associated to genetically predisposed or immunocompromised dogs. It can be localised or generalised (juvenile and adult).

Clinical signs

- Erythema, alopecia, comedones.
- Scabs and furunculosis.
- Limited to the extremities: pododemodicosis.

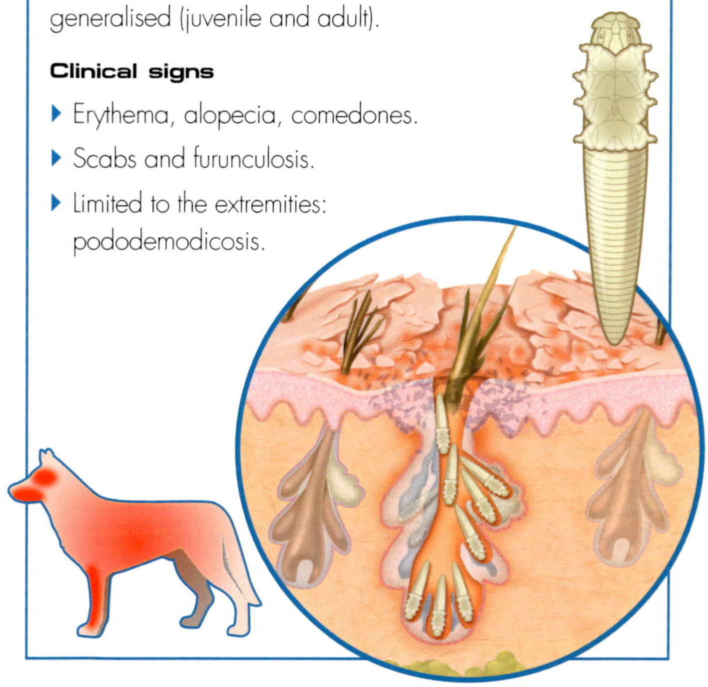

Otodectic mange*

The mite *Otodectes cynotis* is located in the external ear canal. It is more frequent in puppies.

Clinical signs

- Otitis (with secondary bacterial infections).
- Dark ear wax.
- Pruritus.

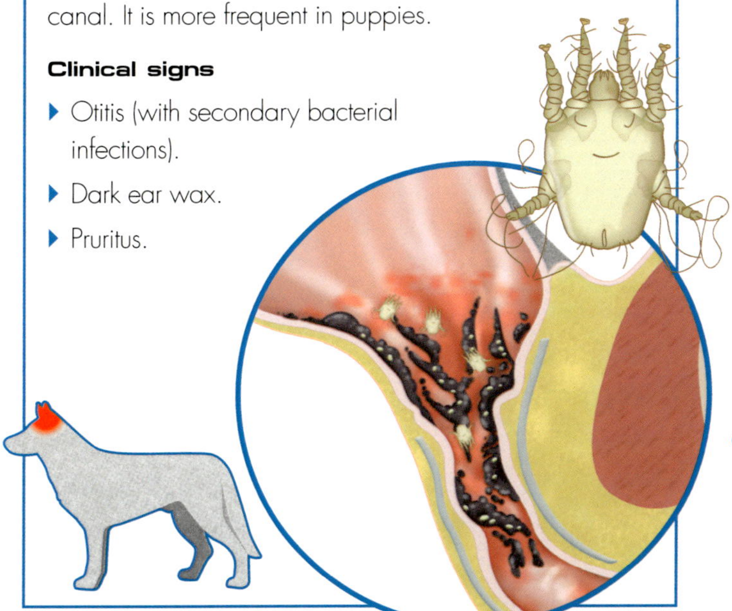

Cheyletiellosis

Caused by mites of the genus *Cheyletiella*. They are located on the skin, not burrow galleries.

Clinical signs

- Pruritus (excoriations).
- Scaling.
- Alopecia.

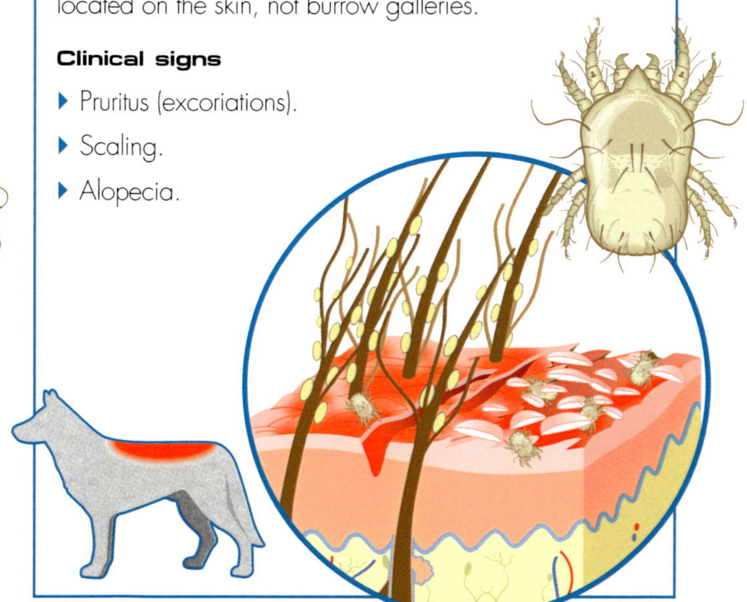

* Infection to people is extremely rare.

SKIN AND ADNEXA

34 Fungal and yeast infections

Dermatophytosis

Caused by fungi *Microsporum*, *Trichophyton*, or *Epidermophyton*. Infection occurs through contact with infected animals. Predisposing factors: juvenile or senile age, immunosuppression, high temperature and moisture, and skin trauma.

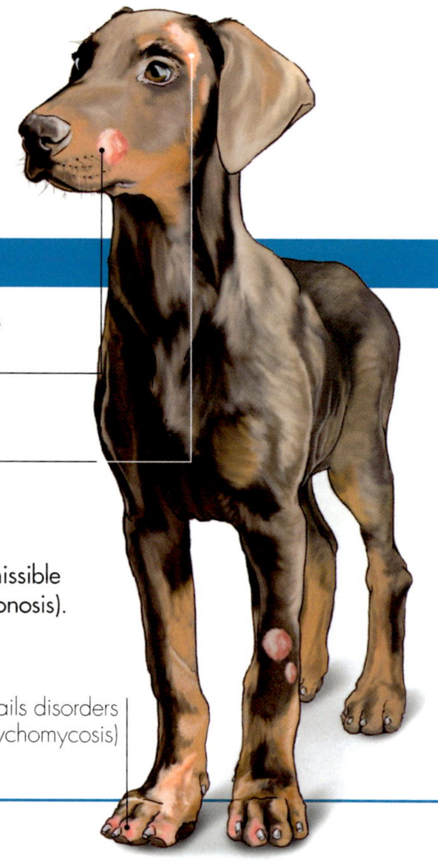

Disease transmissible to humans (zoonosis).

Clinical signs

- Multifocal alopecia and scaling on the face, head and foot region.
- Folliculitis and furunculosis.
- Pruritus.
- Onychomycosis.
- Granulomas.
- Kerion (nodular lesion).

Malassezia pachydermatis dermatitis

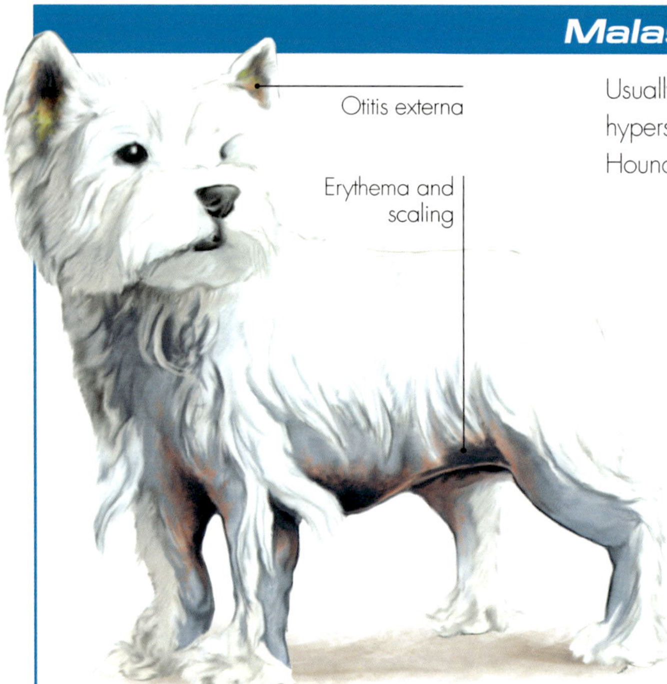

Usually secondary to a disorder that causes overgrowth of yeast and hypersensitivity reactions. There is some breed predisposition in Basset Hound and West Highland White Terrier.

Predisposing factors: changes in immunity, alterations to the cutaneous microclimate and problems in the physiology of the epidermis.

Clinical signs

- Otitis externa: heavy, ceruminous, brown, malodorous discharge.
- Pruritus, erythema, seborrhoea (musty smell).
- Scaling, alopecia, lichenification and hyperpigmentation.

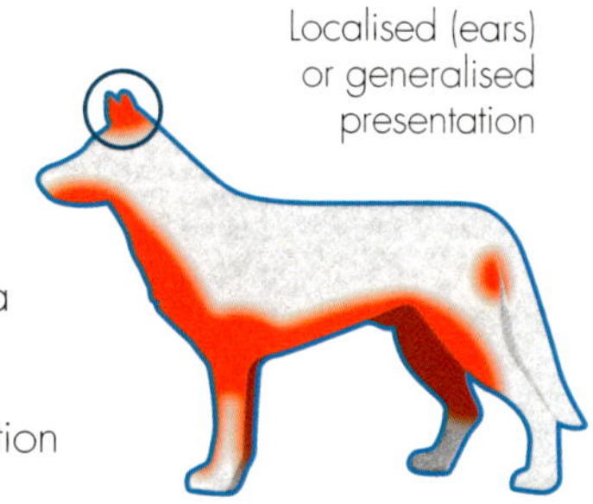

Medical treatment

- Topical therapy: baths and solutions.
- Systemic therapy.

Recommendations

- Cutting hair and disinfecting the environment is advisable in dermatophytosis (diagnosis by ultraviolet light examination and culture).
- Treatment should not be discontinued until at least two negative cultures performed two weeks apart are obtained.

SKIN AND ADNEXA

35 Hypersensitivity

Allergies

Atopic dermatitis

Allergic reaction against environmental antigens which can penetrate through the skin, by inhalation or even swallowed (pollens, moulds, mites, etc.).

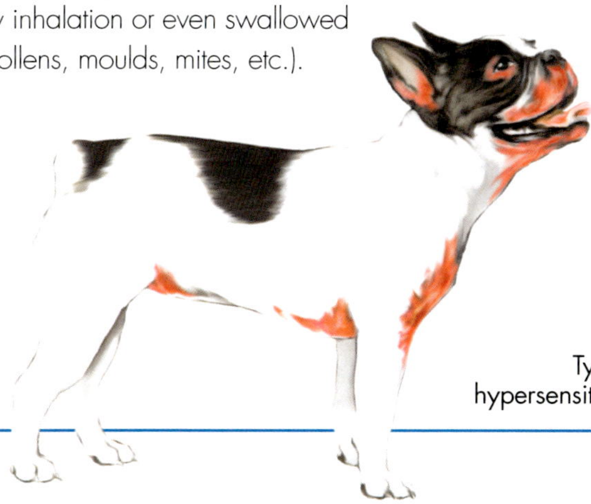

Type I hypersensitivity

Food hypersensitivity

Exaggerated immune response against the ingestion of specific food allergens.

Type I hypersensitivity

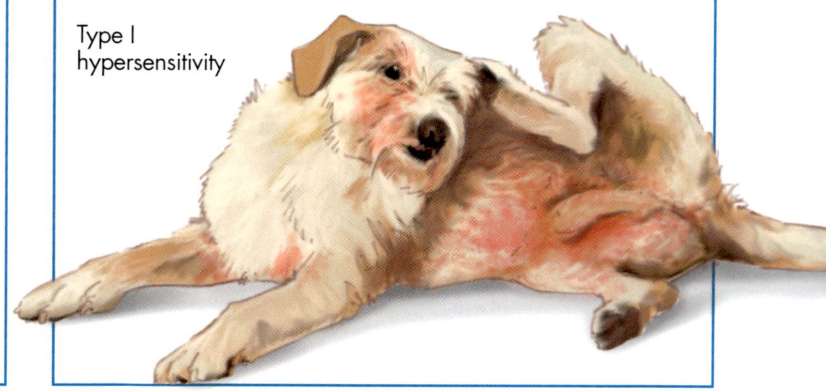

Contact dermatitis (allergic)

Reaction to small amounts of allergens from synthetic materials such as plastics (feeder), textile (bed cover, carpets), collars, hygiene products, plants, etc.

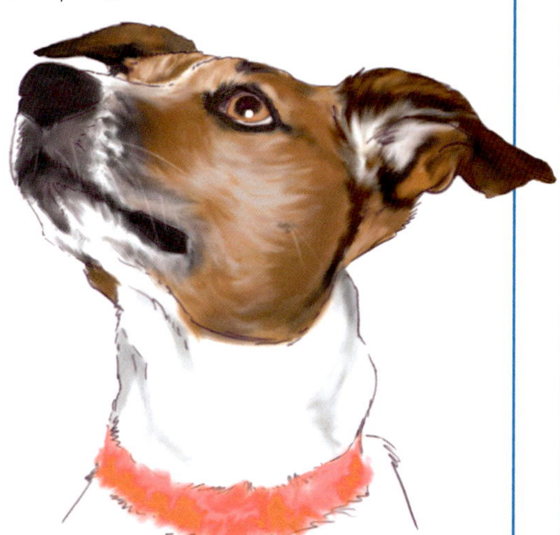

Type IV hypersensitivity

Urticaria and angiooedema

Oedematous process triggered by adverse reactions to food, drugs, insect bites or contact with processionary. Acute or peracute onset.

Type I hypersensitivity

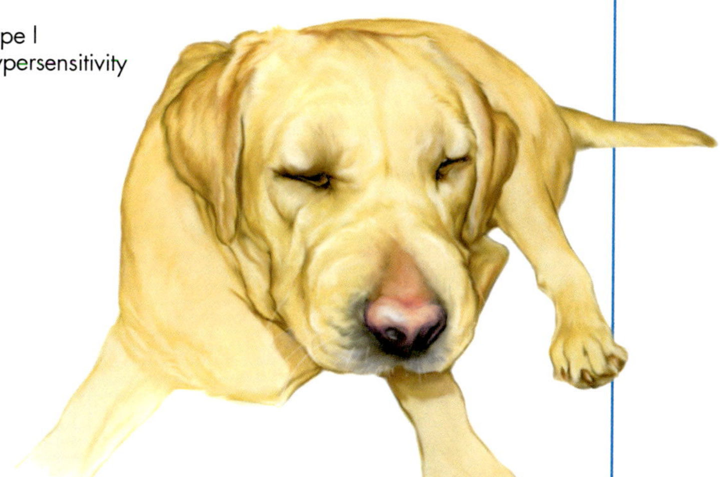

Clinical signs

- Pruritus, erythema, papules, etc.
- Otitis.
- Self-trauma and secondary infection (pyoderma and *Malassezia*).
- Alopecia, hyperpigmentation and lichenification.
- Gastrointestinal problems in food hypersensitivity (10-30 % of cases).

Flea allergy dermatitis is a special type hypersensitivity (late-phase immediate reaction) in which flea saliva is the antigen.

SKIN AND ADNEXA

36 Pyotraumatic dermatitis

Hot spot

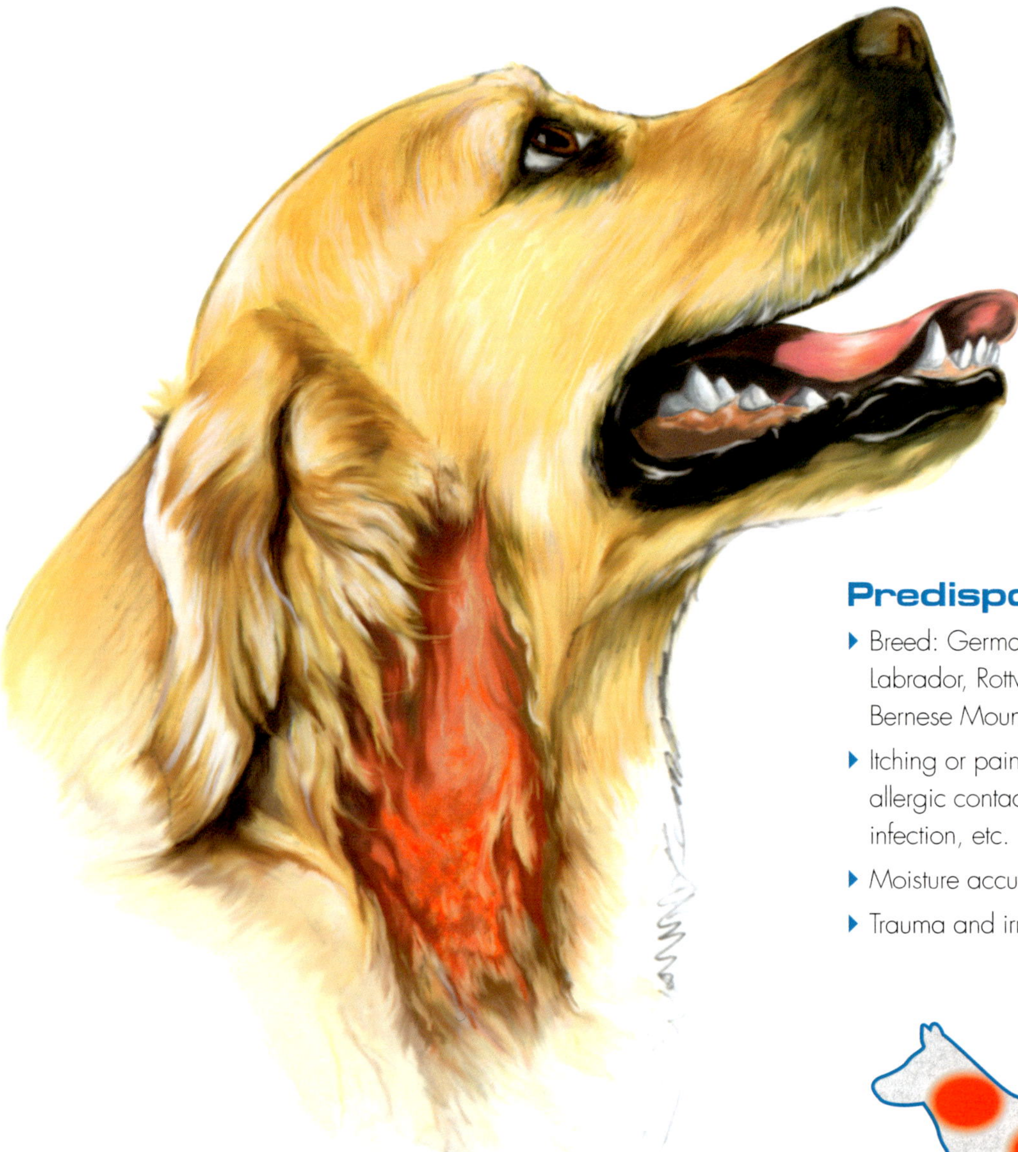

Inflammatory and exudative skin lesion of sudden onset. Self-induced by scratching, licking and rubbing due to the pain or pruritus suffered by the dog.

Predisposing factors

- Breed: German Shepherd, Golden Retriever, Labrador, Rottweiler, Newfoundland, Saint Bernard, Bernese Mountain Dog.
- Itching or pain: allergic disorders (atopic dermatitis, allergic contact dermatitis, FAD), otitis, anal sac infection, etc.
- Moisture accumulation (warm and moist weather).
- Trauma and irritations.

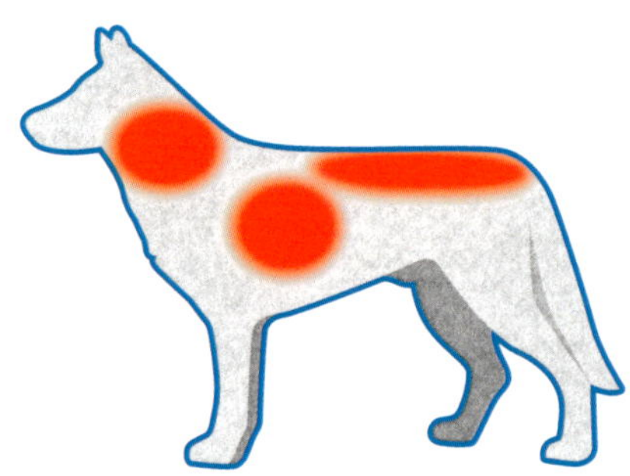

This lesion is easily confused with a wound.

Medical treatment

- Topical: shave the hair and apply antiseptic and anti-inflammatory solutions.
- Systemic: antibiotics and anti-inflammatories.

Clinical signs

- Well-defined lesion of variable size.
- Reddish, moist and exudative skin.
- In dorsal lumbosacral, dorsolateral and periauricular areas.
- Alopecia or coat thickness loss.
- In some occasions, excoriations are observed.

SKIN AND ADNEXA

37 Otitis externa

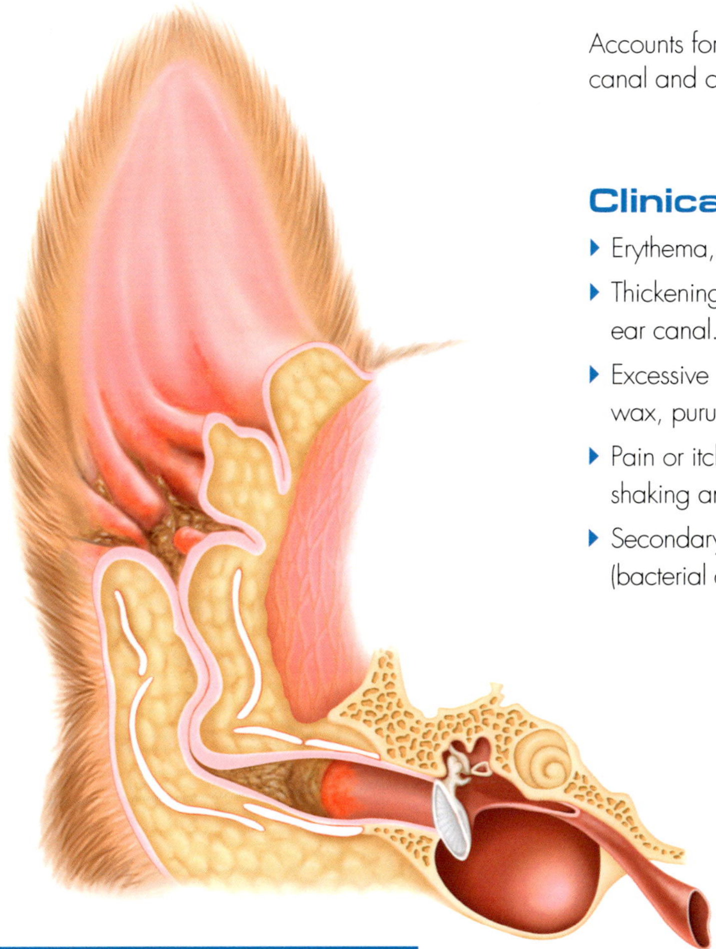

Accounts for 10-20 % of canine skin diseases. Inflammation of the ear canal and often a symptom of another condition (e.g. allergies).

Clinical signs

- Erythema, malodour.
- Thickening of the walls of the ear canal.
- Excessive exudate, dark wax, purulent discharges.
- Pain or itching, head tilt, shaking and scratching.
- Secondary infections (bacterial and *Malassezia*).

Causes

Primary factors

- Hypersensitivities.
- Ectoparasites (*Otodectes*).
- Foreign bodies.
- Autoimmune disorders and keratinization.
- Drug reactions.
- Endocrine diseases.

Predisposing factors

- Conformation (drop eared breeds, Shar Pei).
- Ear canal occlusions (neoplasms or polyps).
- Temperature, moisture, lifestyle (dogs swimming).

Ear cleaning

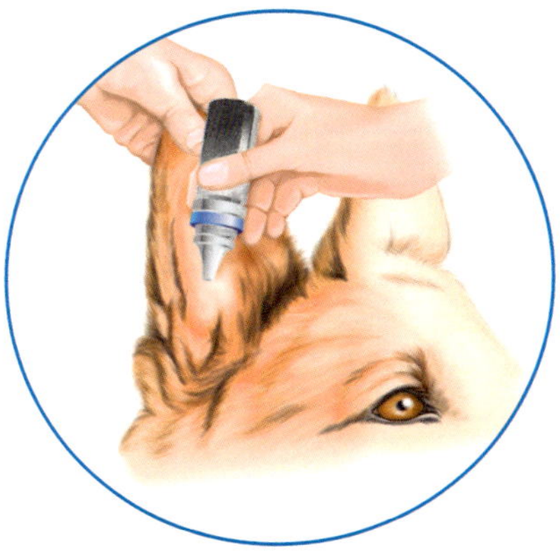

Pulling ear upward to deposit the cleaning liquid.

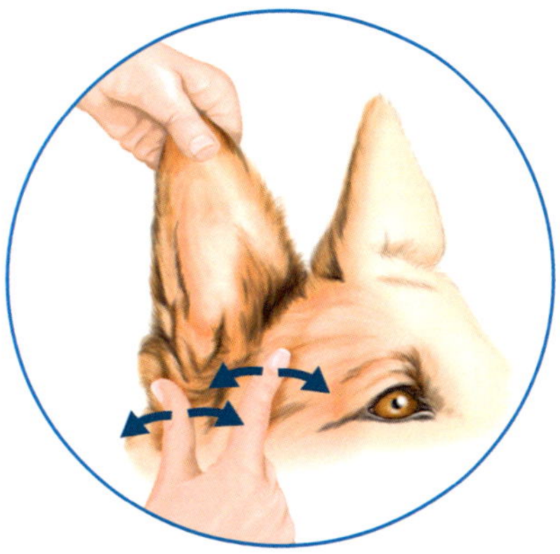

External massage for a few minutes for allowing the product to act.

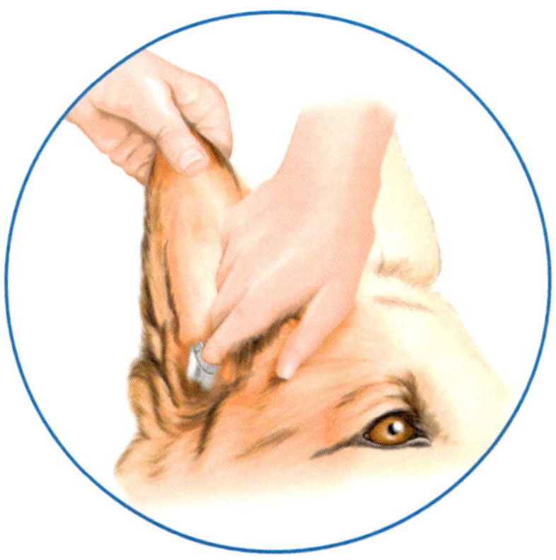

Removing remains of cleanser, dirt and wax with a gauze.

Medical treatment

- Cleaning the ear canal with suitable products.
- Otic drugs to treat the cause: anti-inflammatory, antibacterial, antiparasitic and antifungal.
- Treating the primary cause.

SKIN AND ADNEXA

38 Impetigo and juvenile cellulitis

Impetigo (superficial pyoderma)

Bacterial infection that usually affects puppies a few months old. Appears on hairless areas such as groins, armpits and abdomen and is characterised by the presence of pustules.

It may be due to nutritional causes, parasitoses (immunosuppression) or poor breeding conditions (lack of hygiene in the affected areas).

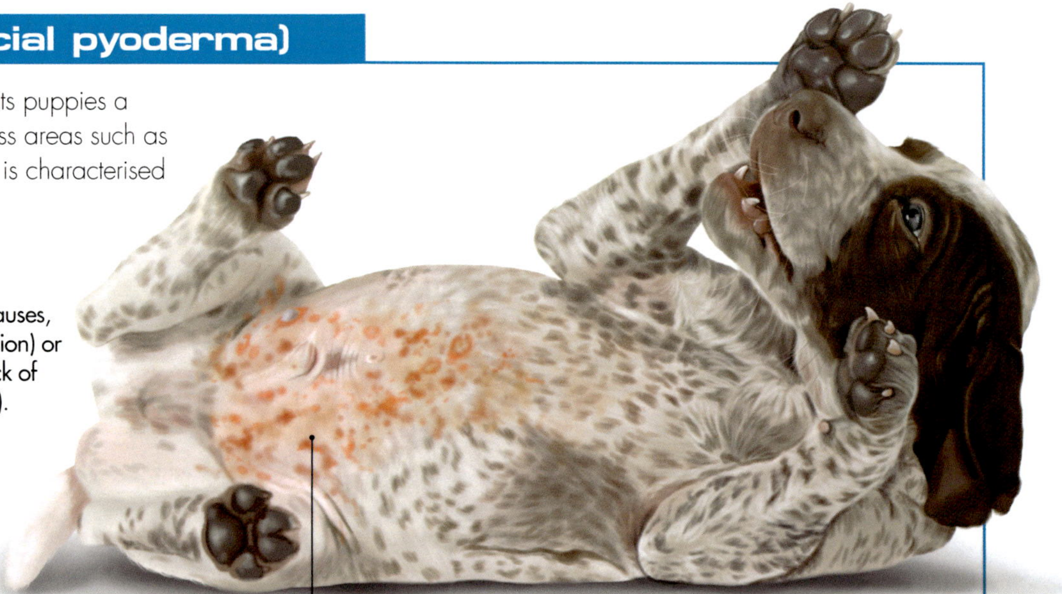
Pustules and epidermal collarettes (annular lesion remains when a pustule breaks)

Juvenile cellulitis (juvenile pyoderma)

Pustular and granulomatous disorder that affects the face, ears and submandibular lymph nodes of puppies and it may be accompanied by fever. Immune alteration is suspected.

More frequent in Labrador, Golden Retriever and Dachshund breeds.

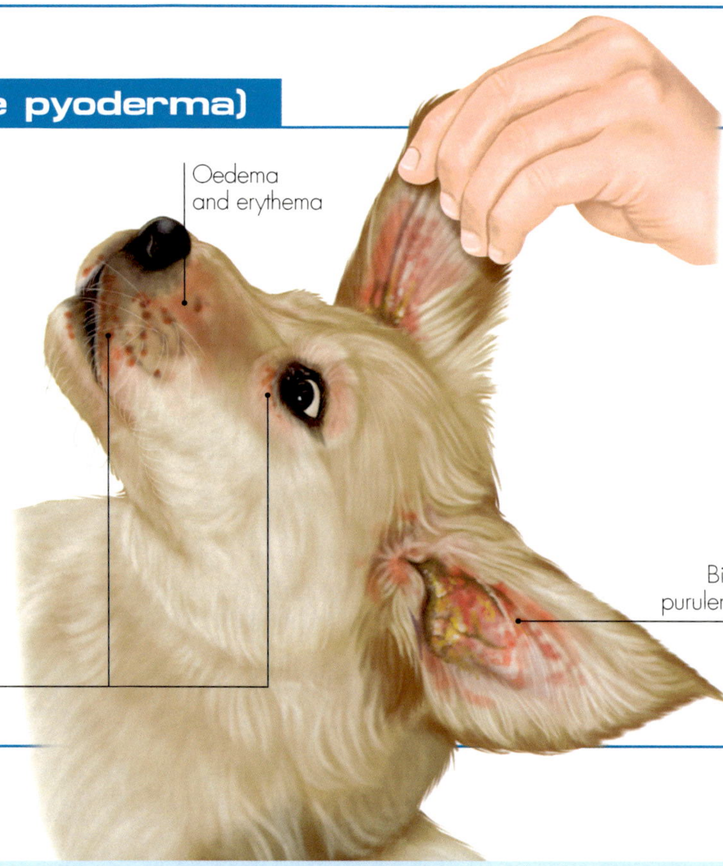

Medical treatment

Impetigo:
- Chlorhexidine baths (every 1-2 days).
- Topical antiseptics (povidone iodine).

Juvenile cellulitis:
- Immunosuppresive drugs and antibiotics.

DIGESTIVE

39 Dental anatomy of the dog

Deciduous and permanent teeth

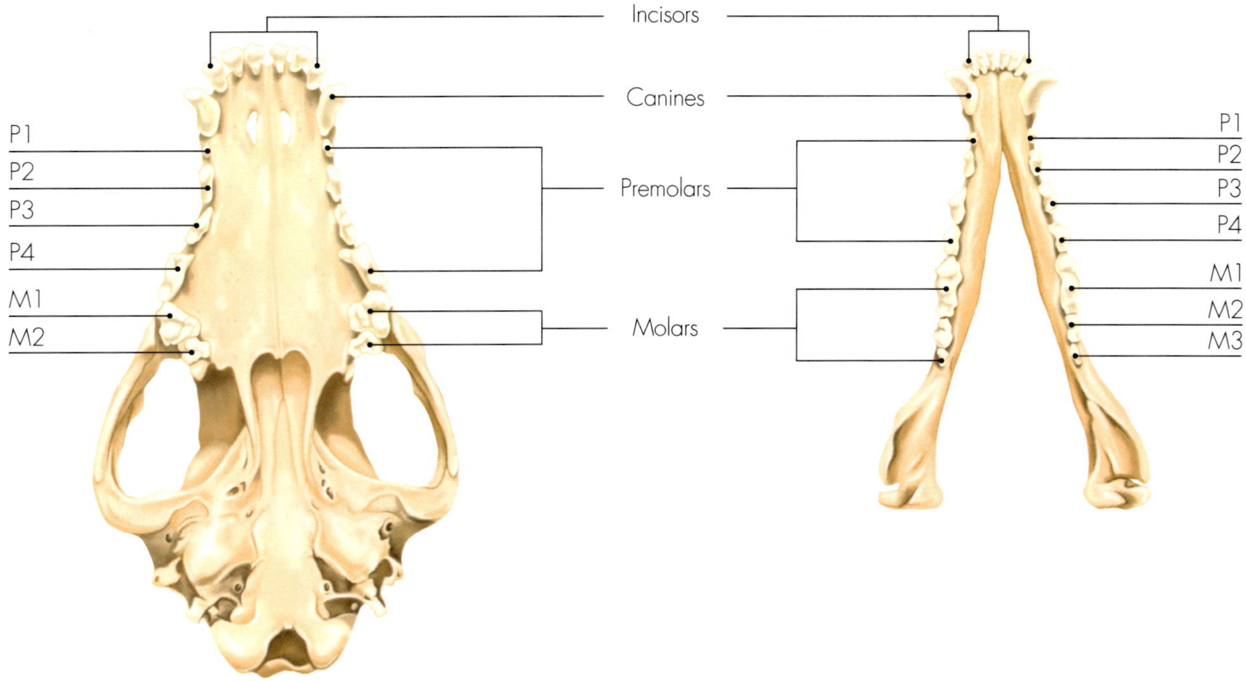

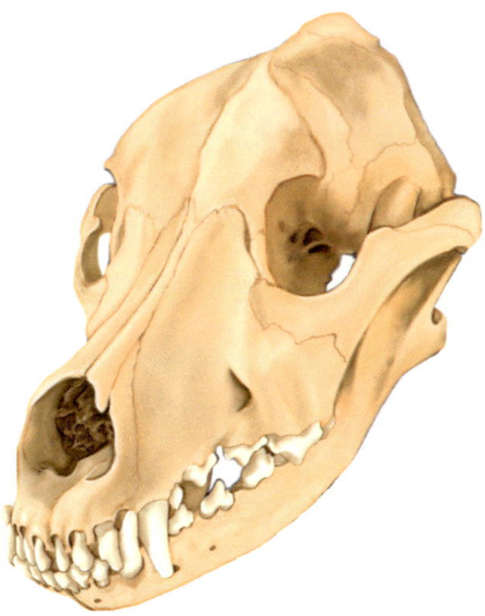

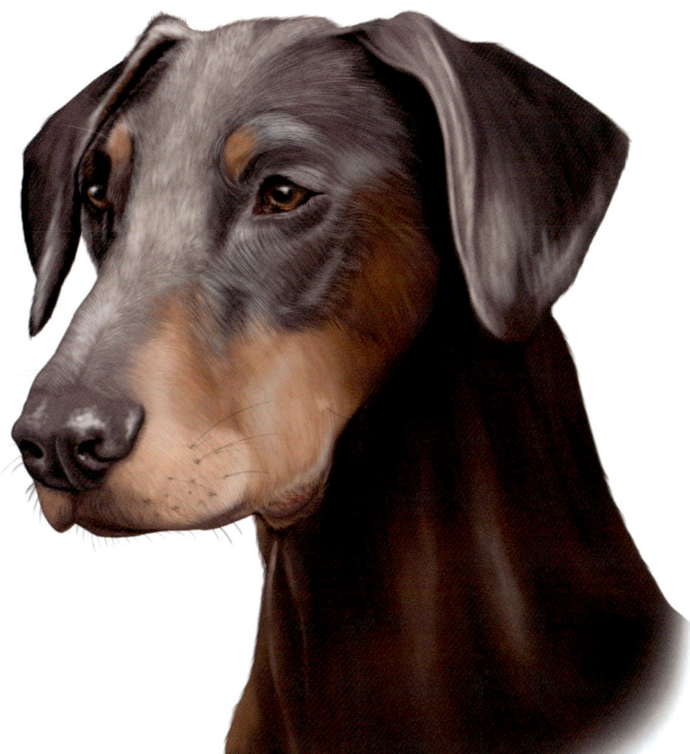

ERUPTION OF DECIDUOUS TEETH IN THE DOG

- **Onset of eruption:** 20 - 30 days
- **End of eruption:** 1.5 - 2 months
- **Fall of deciduous:** 3 - 4.5 months

ERUPTION OF PERMANENT TEETH IN THE DOG*

- **Incisors:** 3 - 4 months
- **Canines:** 4 - 4.5 months
- **1st premolar:** 3.5 - 5 months
- **2nd and 3rd premolar:** 5 months
- **4th premolar:** 4.5 - 6 months
- **1st molar:** 4.5 - 5.5 months
- **2nd molar:** 5 - 7 months
- **3rd molar:** 6 - 7.5 months

* Eruption is later in dwarf and toy breeds than in medium and large breeds.

DENTAL FORMULA OF THE DOG

Deciduous teeth	Permanent teeth
$2 \times \left(I \frac{3}{3}\ C \frac{1}{1}\ P \frac{3}{3} \right) = 28$	$2 \times \left(I \frac{3}{3}\ C \frac{1}{1}\ P \frac{4}{4}\ M \frac{2}{3} \right) = 42$

DIGESTIVE

40 Periodontal disease

The accumulation of dental plaque and calculus (tartar) also affects the surrounding tissues, causing from mild gingivitis to tooth loss, and even serious infections affecting other body organs. It is very common in small and toy breeds from 2 years old.

It may cause oronasal fistulas and mandibular fractures in very advanced stages.

Grades of periodontal disease

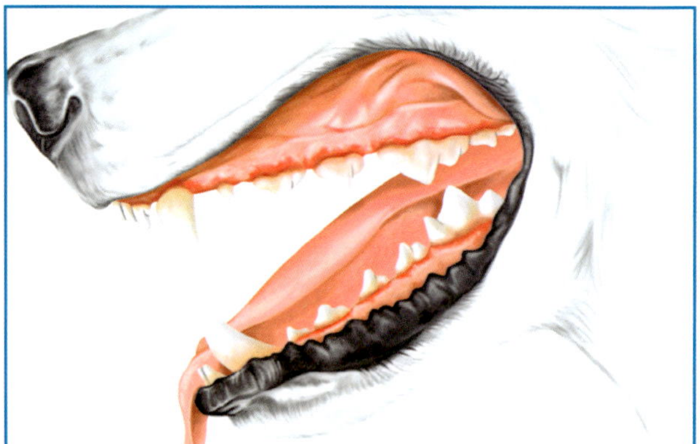

GRADE I: gingivitis

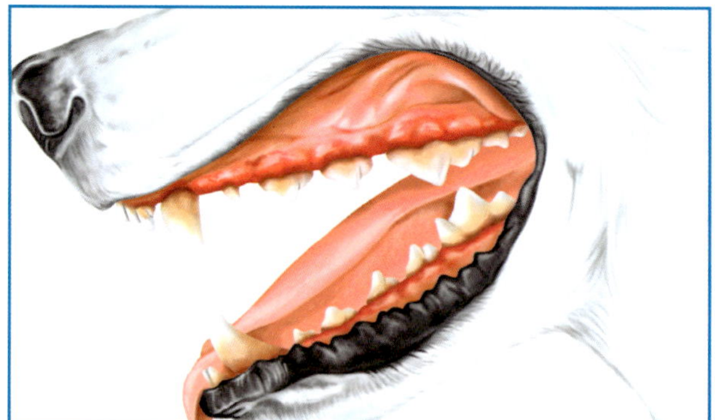

GRADE II: mild periodontitis and periodontal attachment loss <25 %

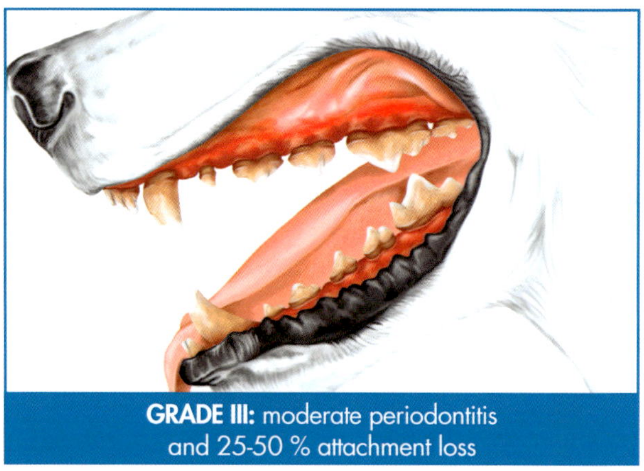

GRADE III: moderate periodontitis and 25-50 % attachment loss

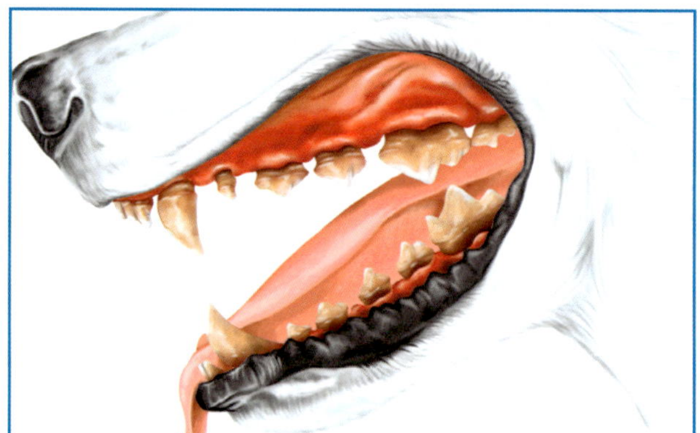

GRADE IV: severe periodontitis and attachment loss

Clinical signs

- Bad breath.
- Gingivitis, bleeding gums.
- Pain, difficulty biting and eating.
- Apathy, behavioural changes.
- Tooth mobility and lack of teeth.

If untreated, periodontal abscesses can be formed, spreading the infection via blood to the heart, liver and kidneys.

Medical treatment

Dental cleaning and systemic treatment (antibiotics).

Surgical treatment

Extraction of the affected teeth may be required.

Recommendations

Prevention by:

- Proper diet.
- Brushing teeth regularly at home.
- Regular dental cleanings by the vet.

DIGESTIVE

41 Main diseases of the oesophagus

The oesophagus connects the oropharyngeal cavity to the stomach. In 90 % of patients having pathologies are described herein.

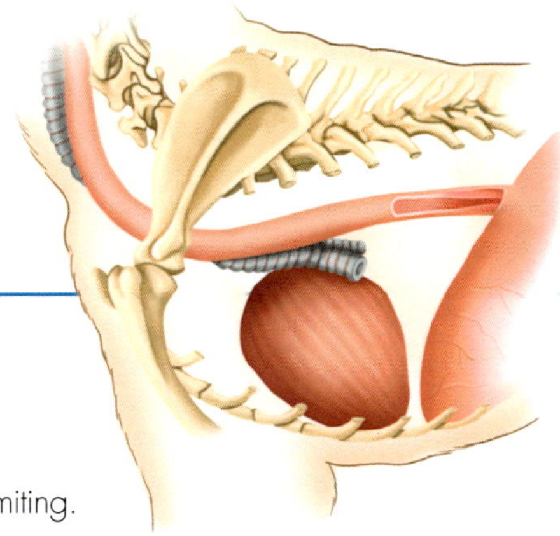

Oesophagitis

- Acute or chronic inflammation of the oesophagus, according to the severity.
- **Causes:** corrosive substances, foreign bodies, persistent vomiting, infections, gastroesophageal reflux, etc.
- **Clinical signs:** difficulty and pain on swallowing, hypersalivation, anorexia, vomiting.

Oesophageal stricture

- Narrowing of the oesophageal duct by a fibrotic inflammatory reaction.
- Any severe damage to the oesophagus can cause its stricture.
- Regurgitation (oesophageal content returning to the mouth undigested) is the most important **clinical sign**.

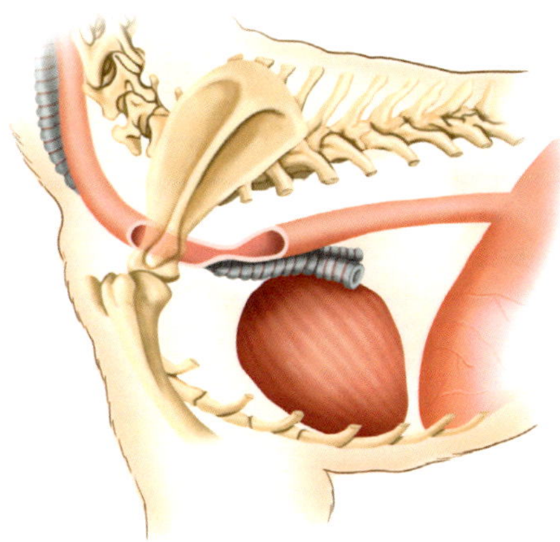

Foreign body

- Ingestion of bones, rubber or cloth toys, hooks, needles, plastics, etc.
- The severity depends on the size and shape of the object and the time it takes hold.

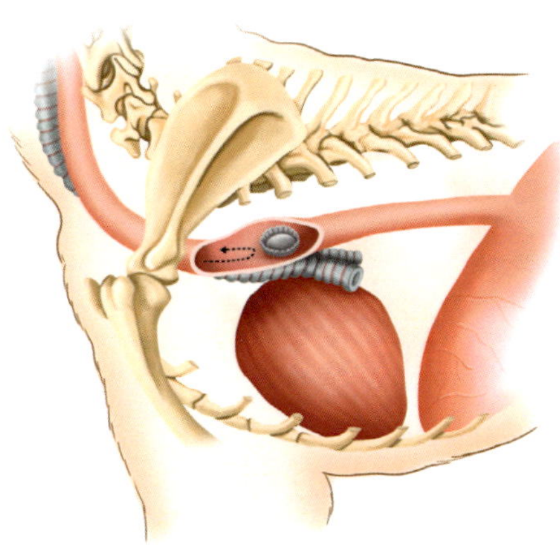

Megaoesophagus

- Generalised dilation of the oesophagus with decreased or total loss of peristalsis.
- It is classified into congenital idiopathic (puppies) and acquired or secondary idiopathic (adults).
- **Main clinical sign**: regurgitation of solid and liquid food by mouth or even nose.

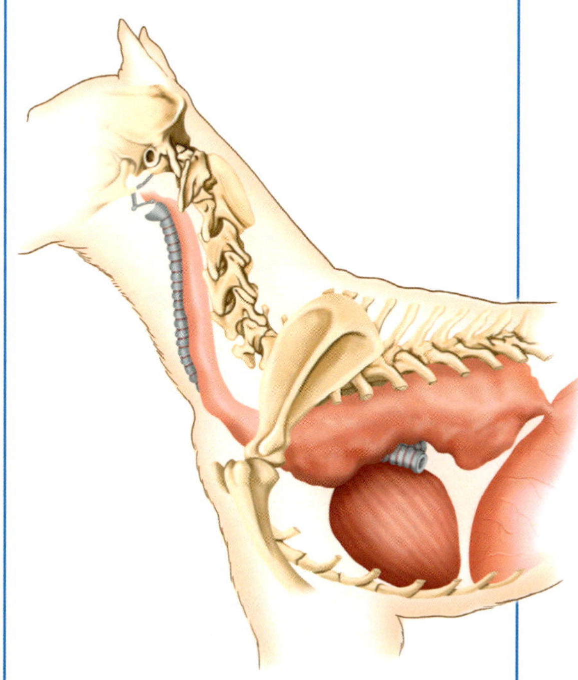

DIGESTIVE

42 Gastric dilation and volvulus syndrome

It appears when the stomach distends and rotates on its longitudinal axis, showing hyperacutely and posing a very serious risk to the dog's life.

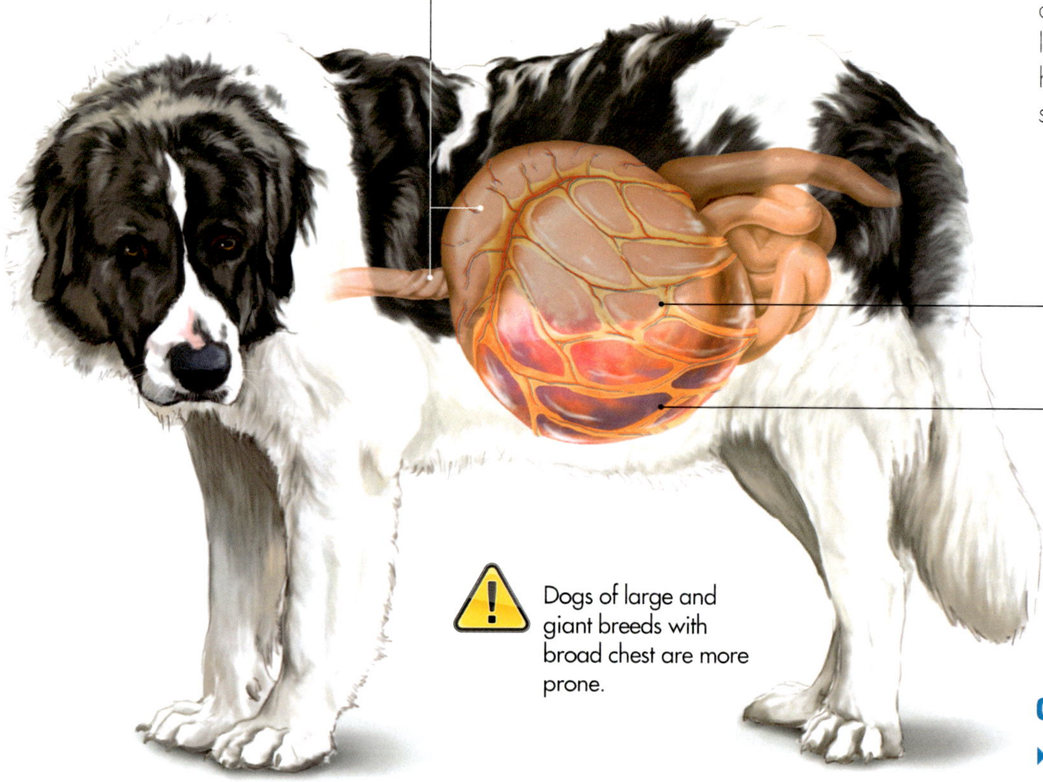
Sphincters (cardia and pylorus) are sealed
The stomach becomes a watertight compartment with accumulation of gas due to the fermentation of the content
Ischaemia and necrosis of the gastric wall

Dogs of large and giant breeds with broad chest are more prone.

Clinical signs

- Restlessness, agitation.
- Salivation, nausea without vomiting.
- Distended abdomen (hollow drum sound).
- Abdominal pain.
- Signs of shock (pallor, weak pulse, etc.).

Triggering factors

- Ingestion of too much food.
- Intense exercise before or after eating.
- Ingestion of large amounts of water after eating.
- Stress.

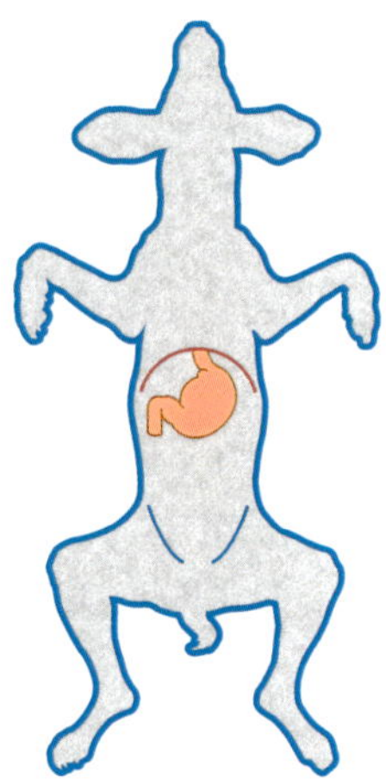

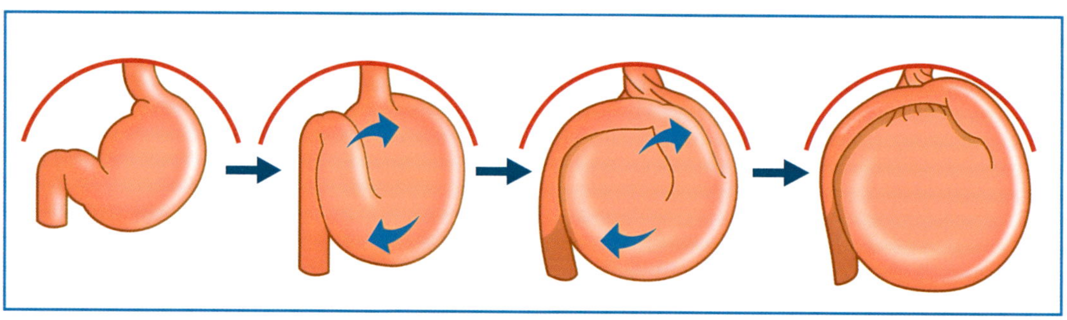

Medical treatment

Introduction of a probe through the mouth to empty the contents of the stomach and subsequent gastric lavage.

Surgical treatment

Surgery for replacement of stomach and spleen, or removal of the spleen and stomach if necrosis has been undergone.

DIGESTIVE

43 Gastrointestinal foreign bodies

These objects, after being ingested, may become lodged in the stomach or intestine due to its size and shape, causing gastrointestinal symptoms. They may even cause total occlusion and perforation of the gastrointestinal tract. It is more frequent in young animals.

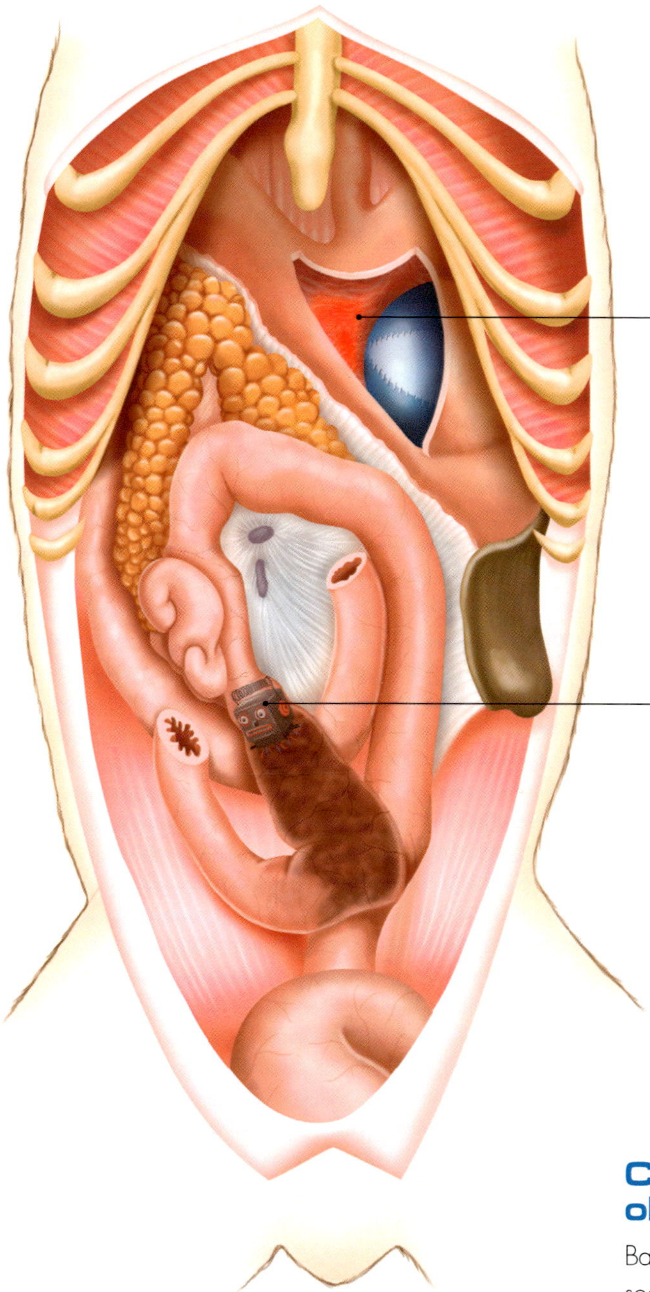

Clinical signs

- Nausea and vomiting.
- Anorexia.
- Lethargy.
- Liquid ileus (decreased peristalsis with fluid accumulation before the foreign body).
- Abdominal pain.
- Signs of shock (due to total occlusion or perforation).

Radiographs, with or without contrast, and ultrasound (in some occasions) are required for detecting the presence of a foreign body.

Common objects

Balls, rubber toys, bones, rags, socks, bottle caps, ropes, stones, fruit pits, cables, wires, needles, hooks, etc.

Medical treatment

Supportive treatment until the foreign body is expelled.

Surgical treatment

Object removal by endoscopy or surgery.

DIGESTIVE

44 Most common canine intestinal parasites

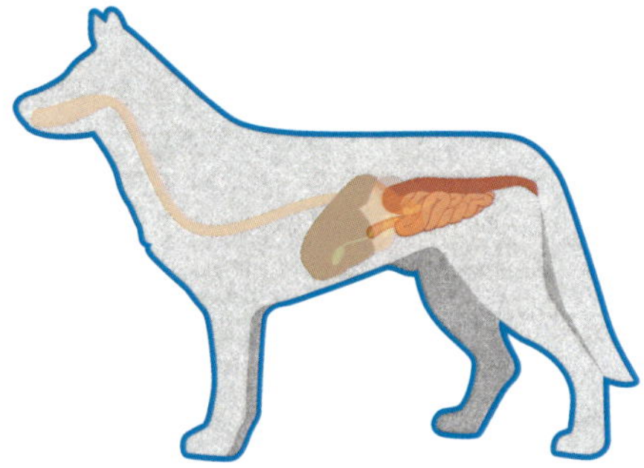

Disease transmissible to humans (zoonosis).

Protozoa

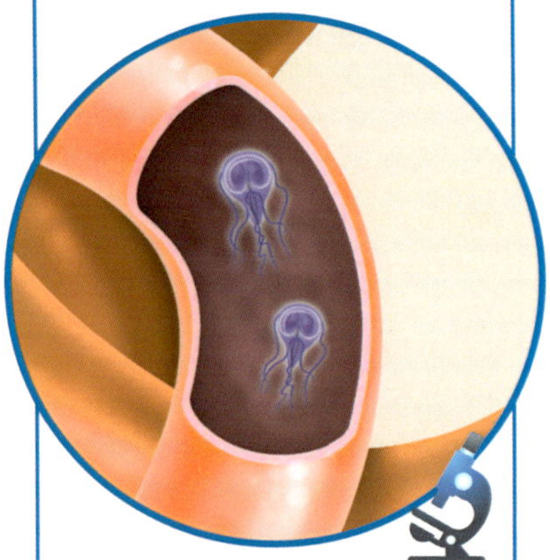

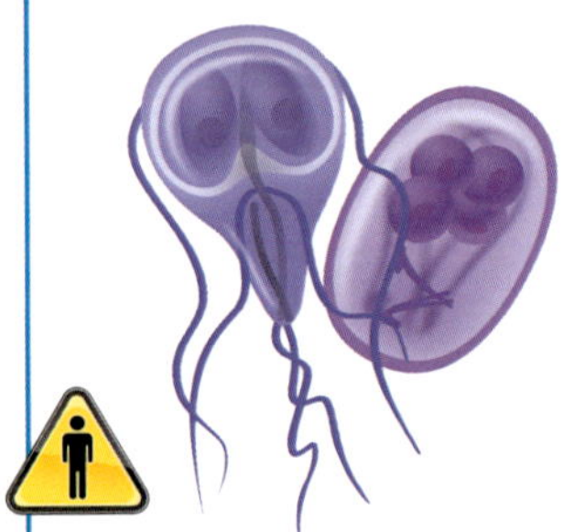

Giardia duodenalis

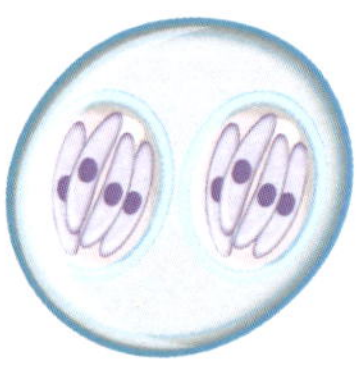

Coccidia (*Cystoisospora*)

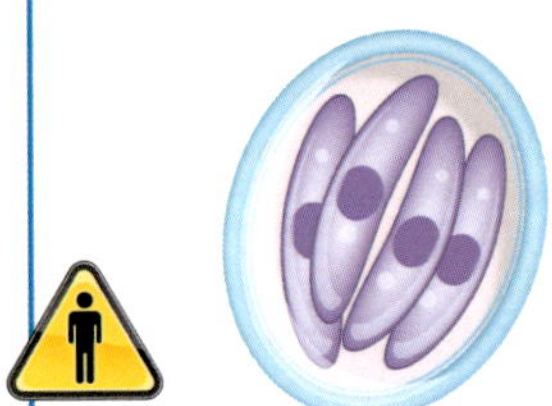

Cryptosporidia (*C. parvum, C. canis*)

Nematodes

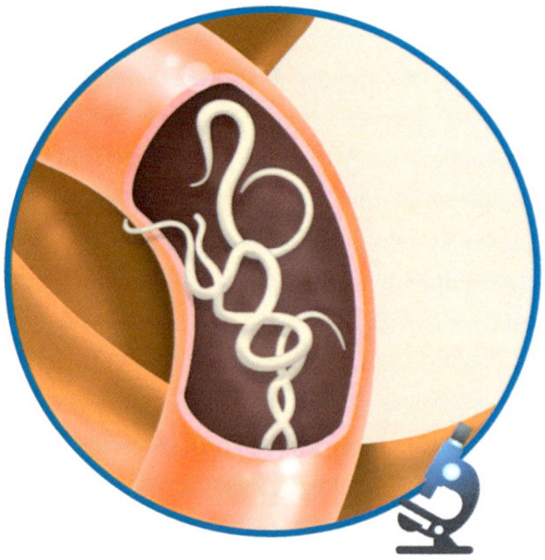

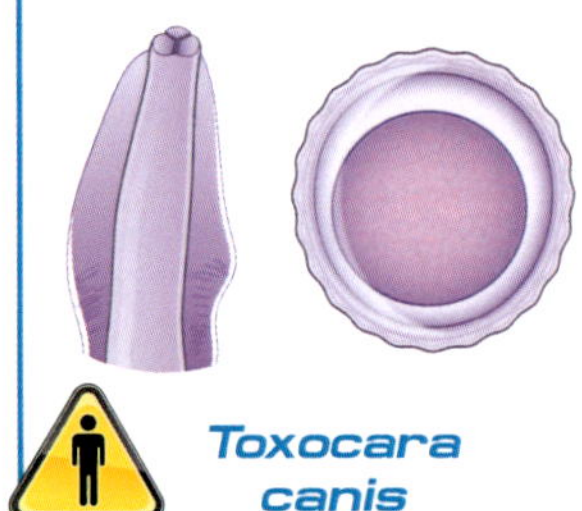

Toxocara canis

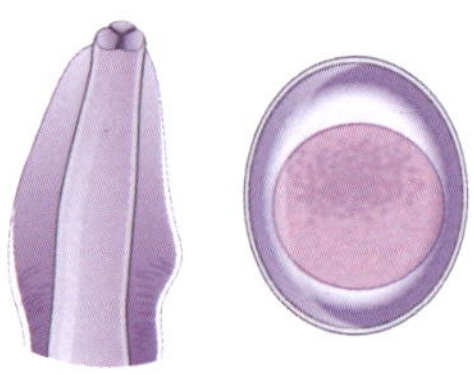

Toxascaris leonina

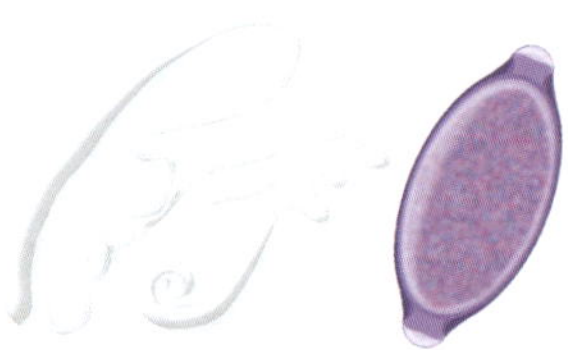

Trichuris vulpis (whipworms)

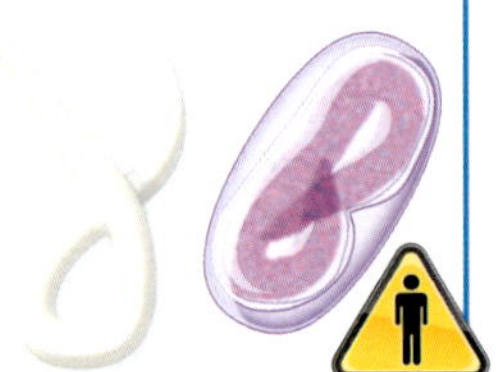

Strongyloides stercoralis

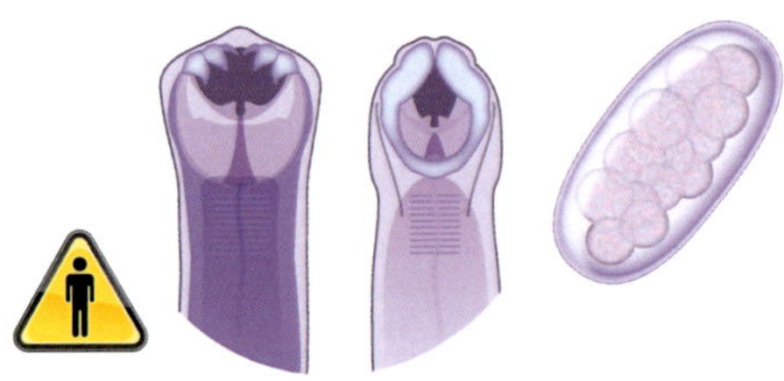

Ancylostoma/Uncinaria (hookworms)

Cestodes

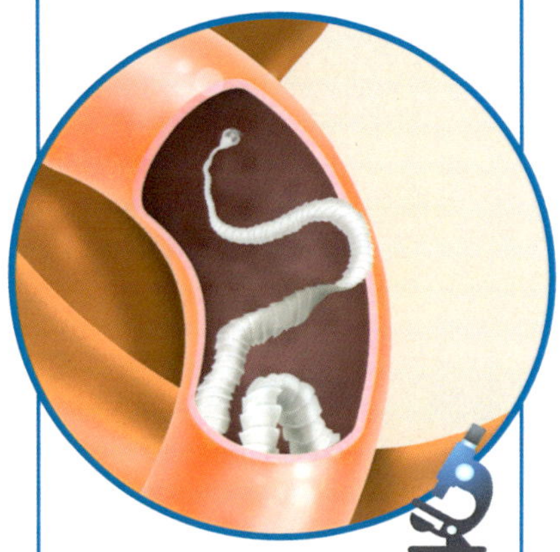

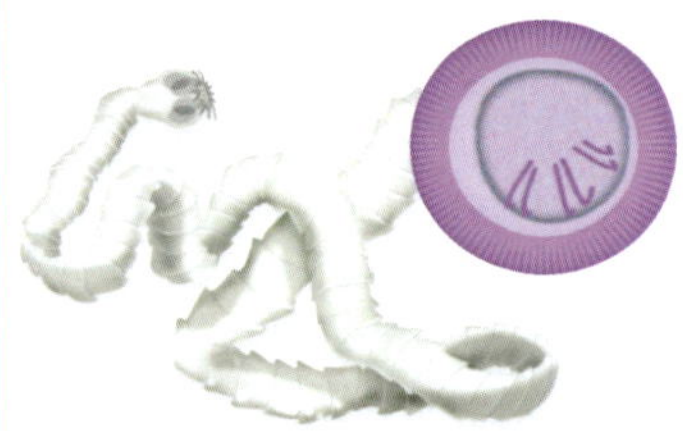

Taenia spp.

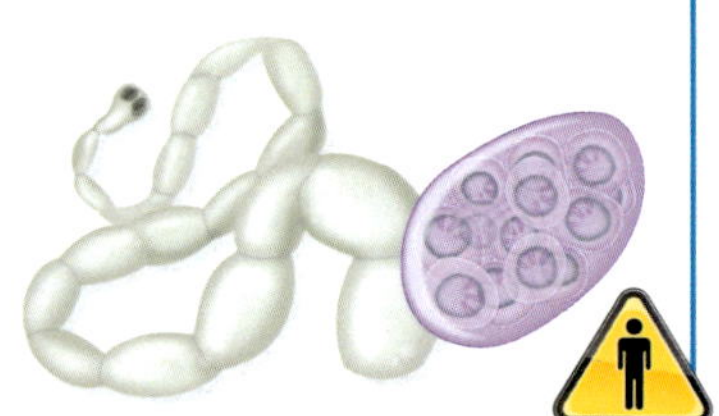

Dypilidium caninum

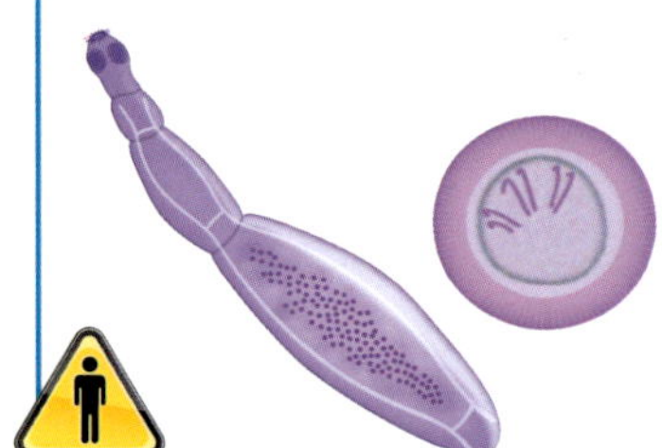

Equinococcus granulosus

DIGESTIVE

45 Pancreatitis and exocrine pancreatic insufficiency

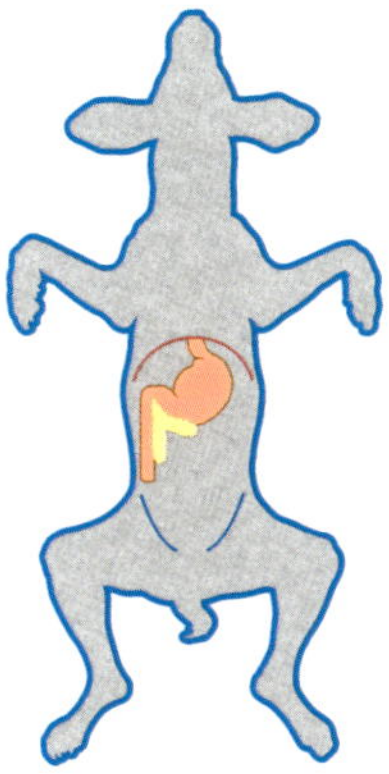

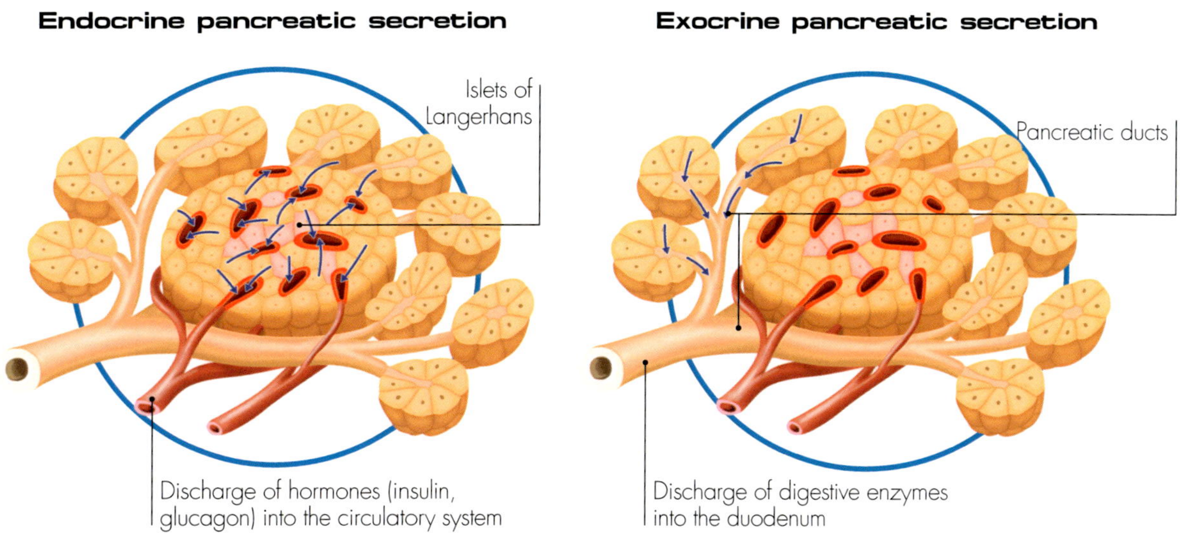

Pancreatitis

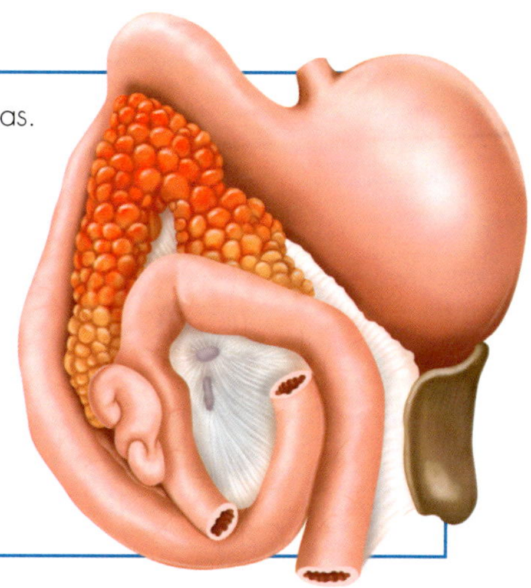

- Acute (reversible) and chronic (irreversible histological changes) inflammation of the pancreas.
- Dogs of middle or advanced age. Schnauzer, Yorkshire Terrier and Poodle are particularly predisposed.
- Possible triggering factors: nutrition (obesity and high-fat diets), certain drugs, infectious diseases, endocrinopathies.

Clinical signs

- Anorexia.
- Vomiting.
- Abdominal pain.
- Dehydration and weakness.
- Diarrhoea.

Exocrine pancreatic insufficiency

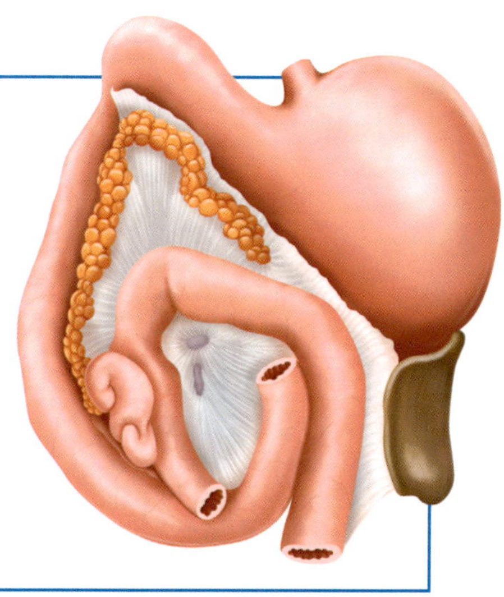

- Destruction of the gland that leads to a maldigestion syndrome due to enzyme deficiency.
- Young dogs (1-4 years), especially German Shepherd, Collie and Chow Chow.
- Most common cause: pancreatic acinar atrophy without involvement of the endocrine pancreas (possible autoimmune origin).
- Treatment: administration of pancreatic enzymes with every meal.

Clinical signs

- Yellow-brownish diarrhoea, very voluminous, with fat and undigested food.
- Bowel sounds and flatulence.
- Poor coat appearance.
- Increased appetite with weight loss.
- Nervousness and aggressiveness.

DIGESTIVE

46 Hepatitis

Inflammation of the liver can follow an acute or chronic course. They are considered chronic if last more than 4-6 months. A loss of liver's capacity to regenerate and fibrosis (cirrhosis) occurs.

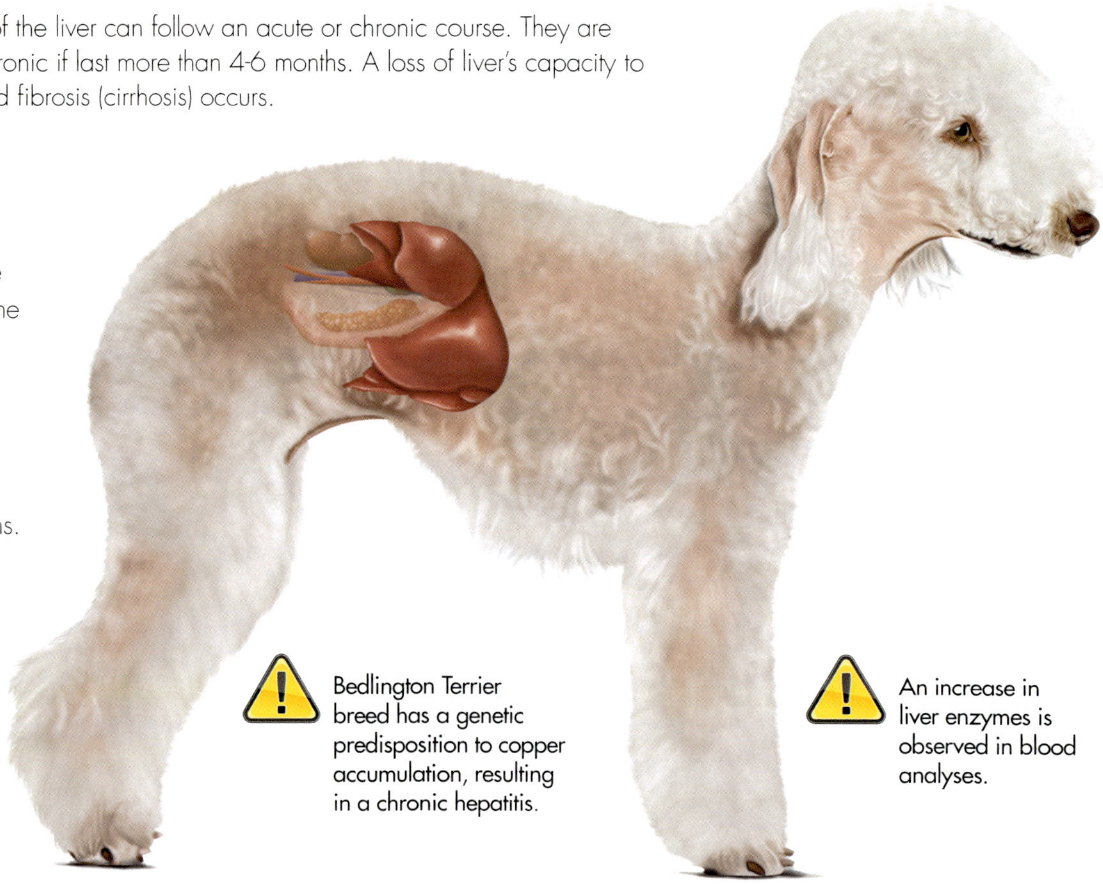

Causes

- Infection: infectious canine hepatitis adenovirus, canine herpesvirus, leptospirosis.
- Toxins.
- Hepatic hypoxia.
- Drugs.
- Immune-mediated reactions.
- Metabolic disorders.
- Copper accumulation.

Bedlington Terrier breed has a genetic predisposition to copper accumulation, resulting in a chronic hepatitis.

An increase in liver enzymes is observed in blood analyses.

Acute hepatitis

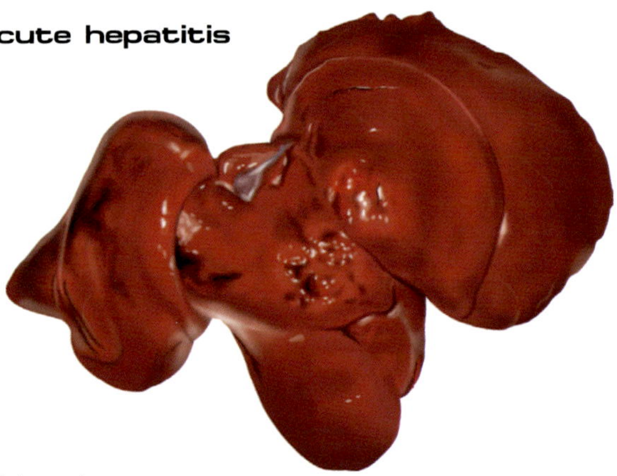

- Enlarged.
- Marked increase in liver enzymes.
- Mild signs of disease.

Chronic hepatitis (cirrhosis)

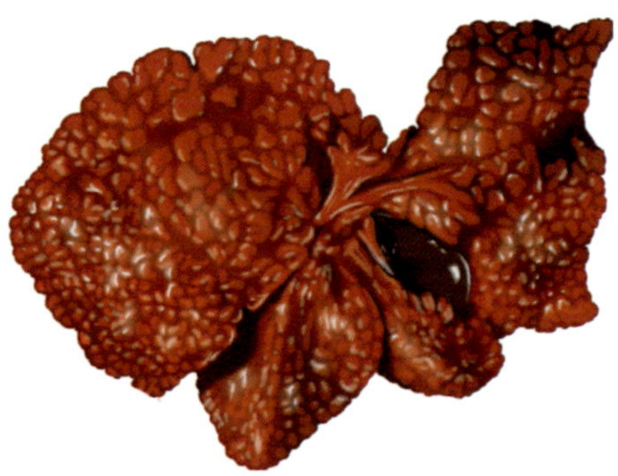

- Decrease in size.
- Moderate increase in liver enzymes.
- Severe signs of disease.

Medical treatment

Counteract the cause, alleviate symptoms and protect the liver.

Clinical signs

- Nonspecific: malaise, lethargy, anorexia, vomiting, dehydration, jaundice, fever, diarrhoea.
- In severe cases: hepatic encephalopathy, DIC, hypoglycaemia, coma and death.

DIGESTIVE

47 Portosystemic shunts

Portosystemic shunts are vascular anomalies that allow the passage of blood from the portal vein into the systemic circulation, bypassing the liver. This entails the passage of toxic substances that could not be metabolised in the liver.

They may have an intrahepatic (large breed) or extrahepatic (small breeds) location, and are classified as congenital or acquired, single or multiple.

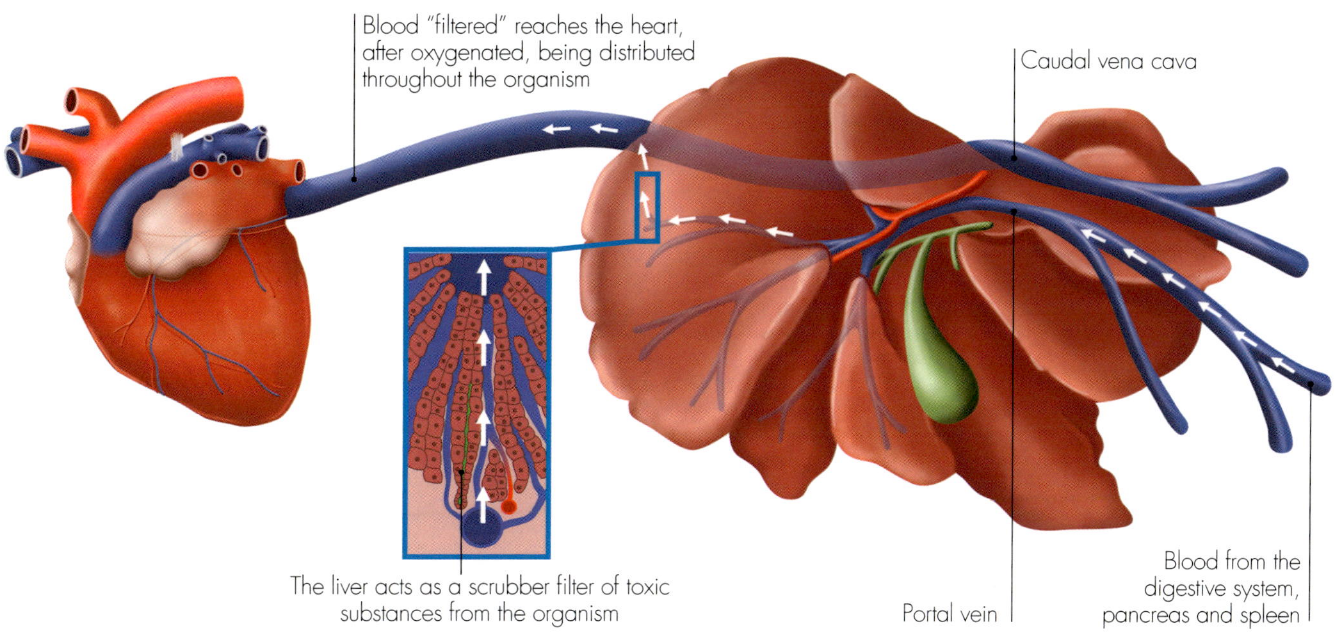

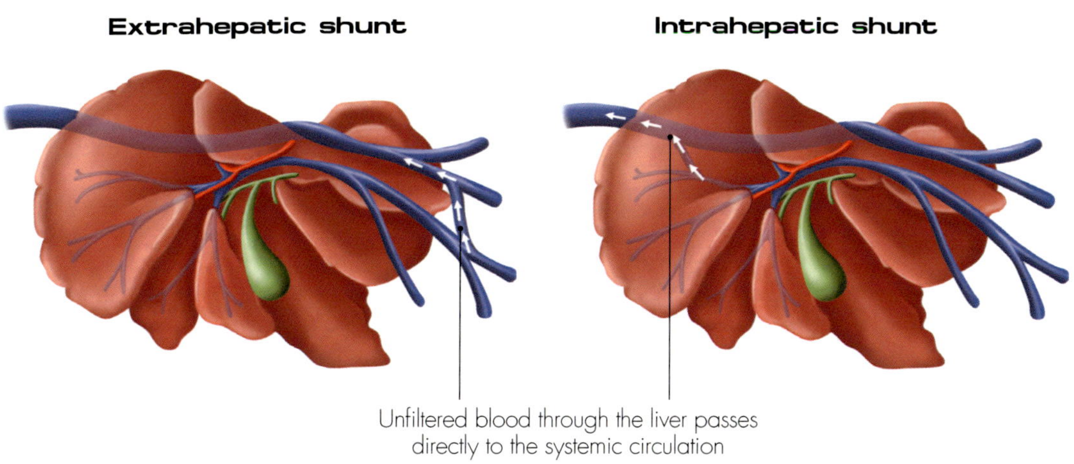

Clinical signs

General

- Poor body condition, small stature (congenital shunt), weight loss (acquired shunt).
- Anorexia.
- Depression, lethargy.

Others

- Neurologic: disorientation, hyperactivity, convulsions, etc.
- Digestive: vomiting, diarrhoea.
- Urinary: haematuria, tenesmus, polyuria and polydipsia, ammonium urate crystals.

Medical / dietary treatment

Alleviate the effects of the accumulation of toxins in the different systems.

Surgical treatment

Partial or total occlusion of the anomalous vessel with techniques such as silk thread ligation, ameroid constrictor band, cellophane, etc.

DIGESTIVE

48 Perinanal disorders

Anal sacculitis: impaction / infection of the anal sacs

- Anal sacs are skin invaginations located on the sides of the anus.
- Its content is removed by compression with defecation and has a characteristic unpleasant odour that may have a social function of recognition and territorial marking.
- Content may be retained, accumulated and become infected (abscess).
- If the problem is not resolved by manual emptying, it gets chronic and may become a fistula.

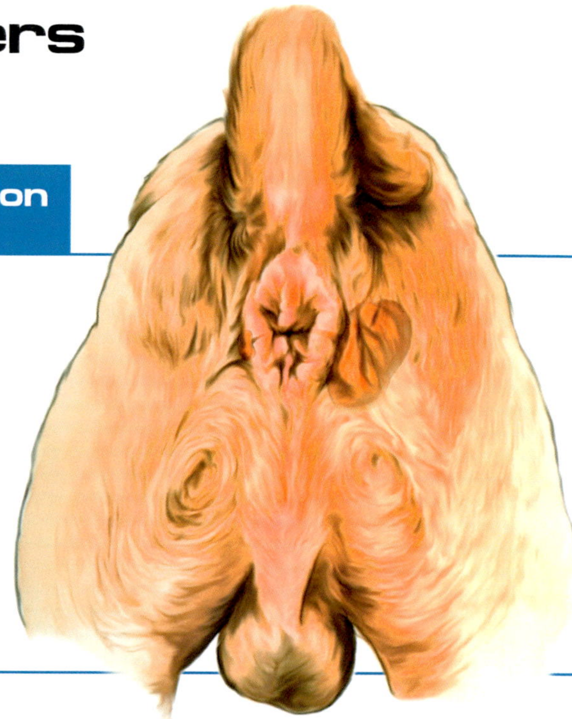

Perianal fistulas

- Progressive chronic condition characterised by ulcerations, fistulas and inflammation of the surrounding tissue.
- They may be associated with anal sacculitis or related to immune-mediated diseases (e.g. reaction to dietary components).

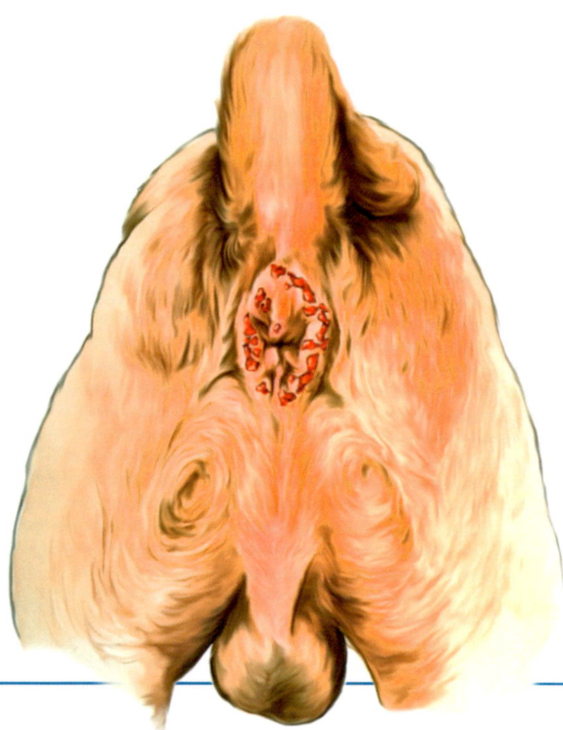

Perianal neoplasias

Specific areas:

- Hepatoid or perianal glands adenoma.
- Hepatoid glands adenocarcinoma.
- Adenocarcinoma of the anal sacs.

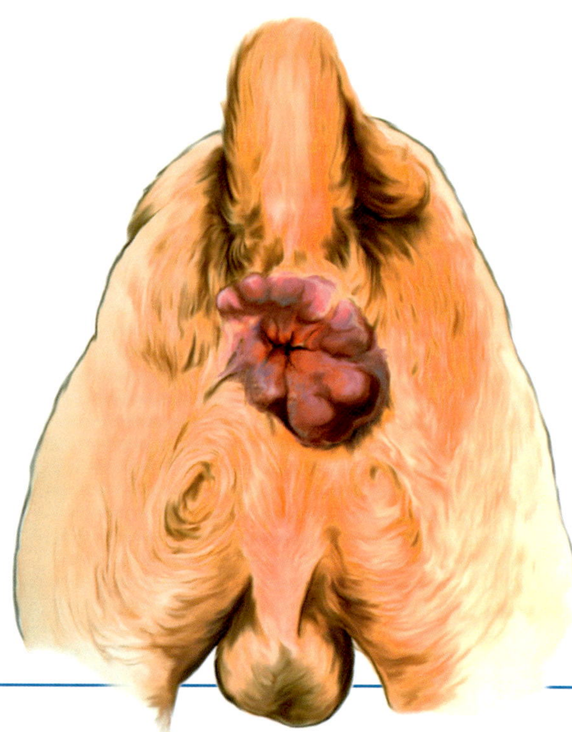

EYES

49 Structures of the eye

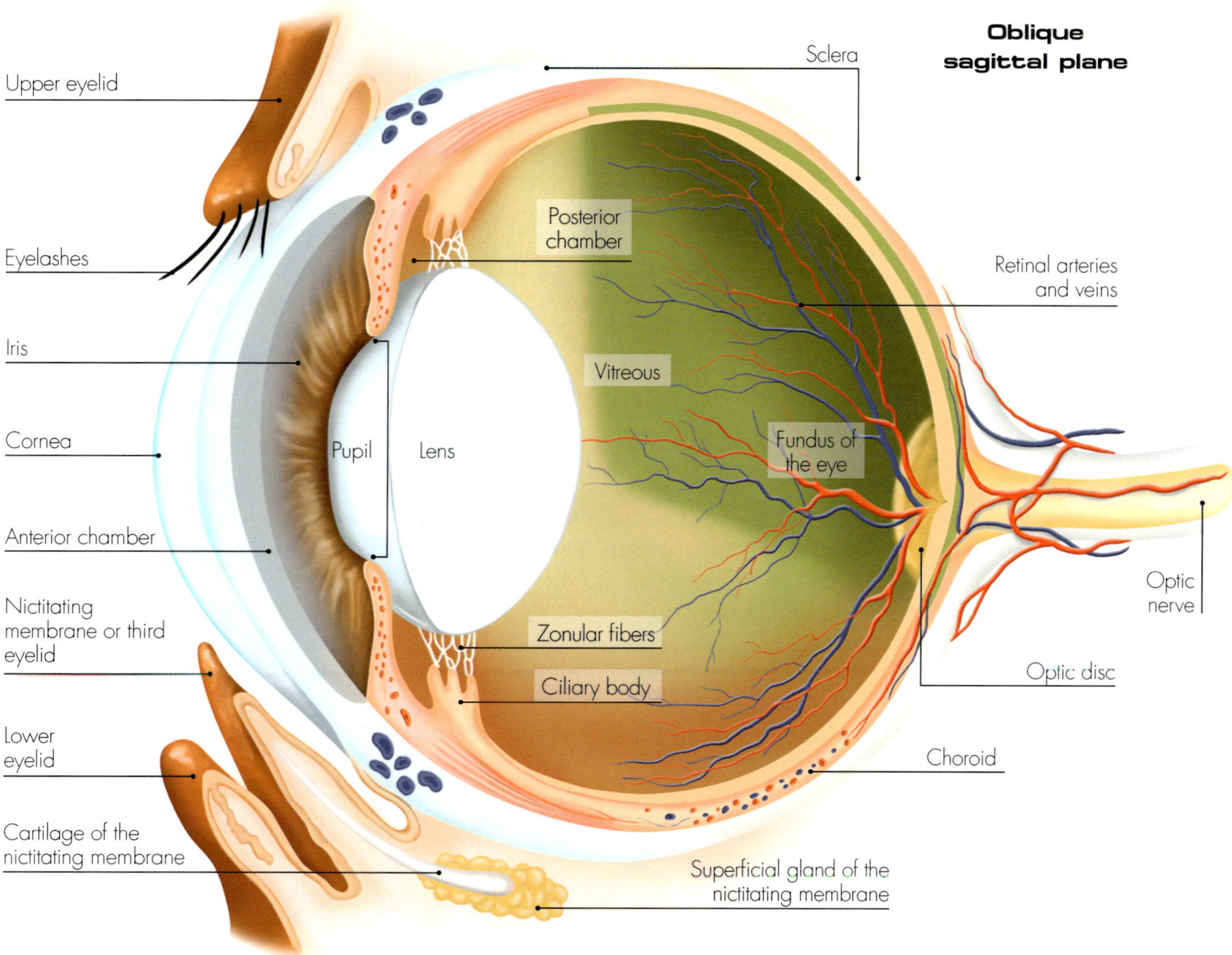

Viewing angle

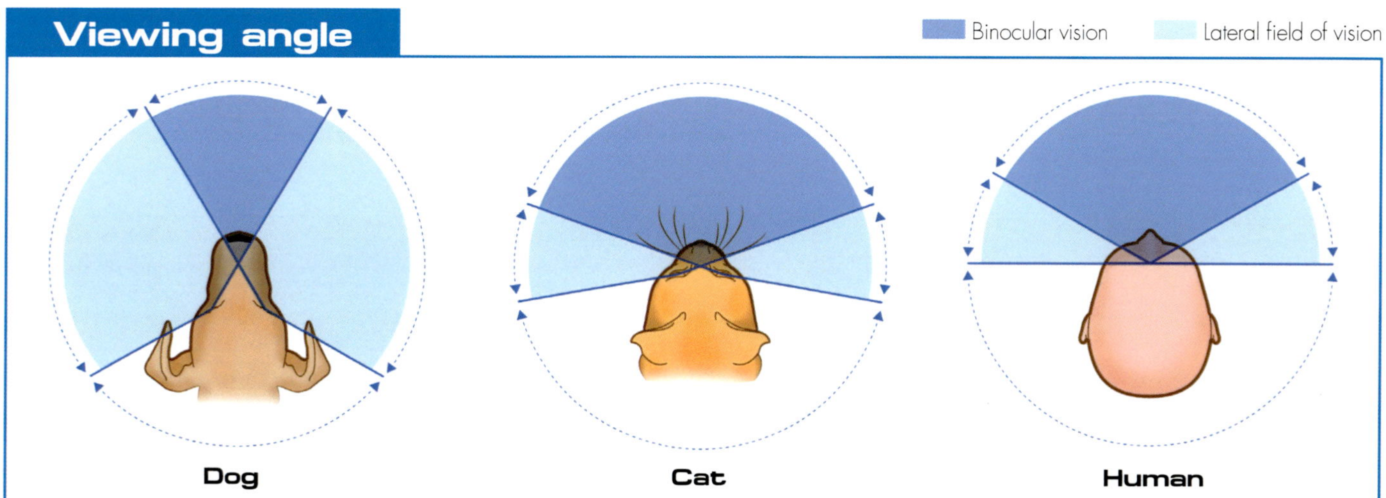

EYES

50 Keratoconjunctivitis sicca (KCS)

Inflammatory disease of the cornea (and conjunctiva) by a deficiency in the quality or quantity of tear film. It may be unilateral or, more often, bilateral. According progresses, the cornea loses its physiological characteristics of transparency, smooth surface, brightness and avascularity.

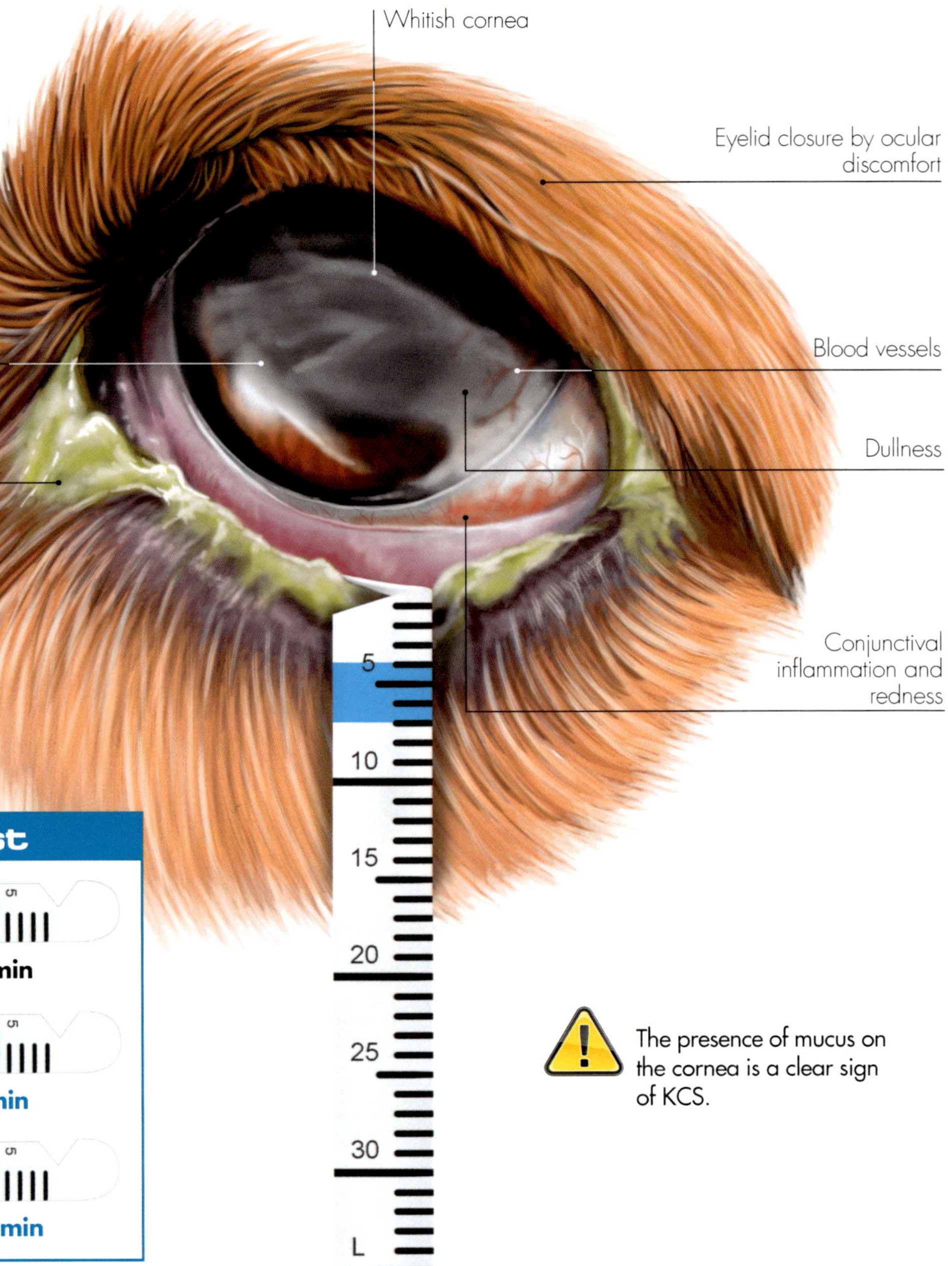

Schirmer's test

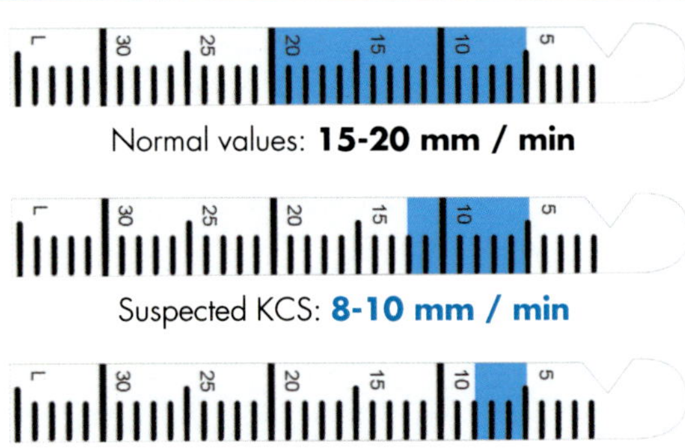

Normal values: **15-20 mm / min**

Suspected KCS: **8-10 mm / min**

Confirmation of KCS: **<8 mm / min**

The presence of mucus on the cornea is a clear sign of KCS.

Medical treatment

- Remove the cause of KCS whenever possible.
- Stimulate tear production or manage tear substitutes.
- Control inflammation and infection.
- Immunosuppressive drugs (cyclosporine) when the source is immune-mediated.

Many KCS have an immune-mediated origin, with involvement of the lacrimal glands (lymphoplasmacytic dacryoadenitis).

EYES

51 Corneal ulcers

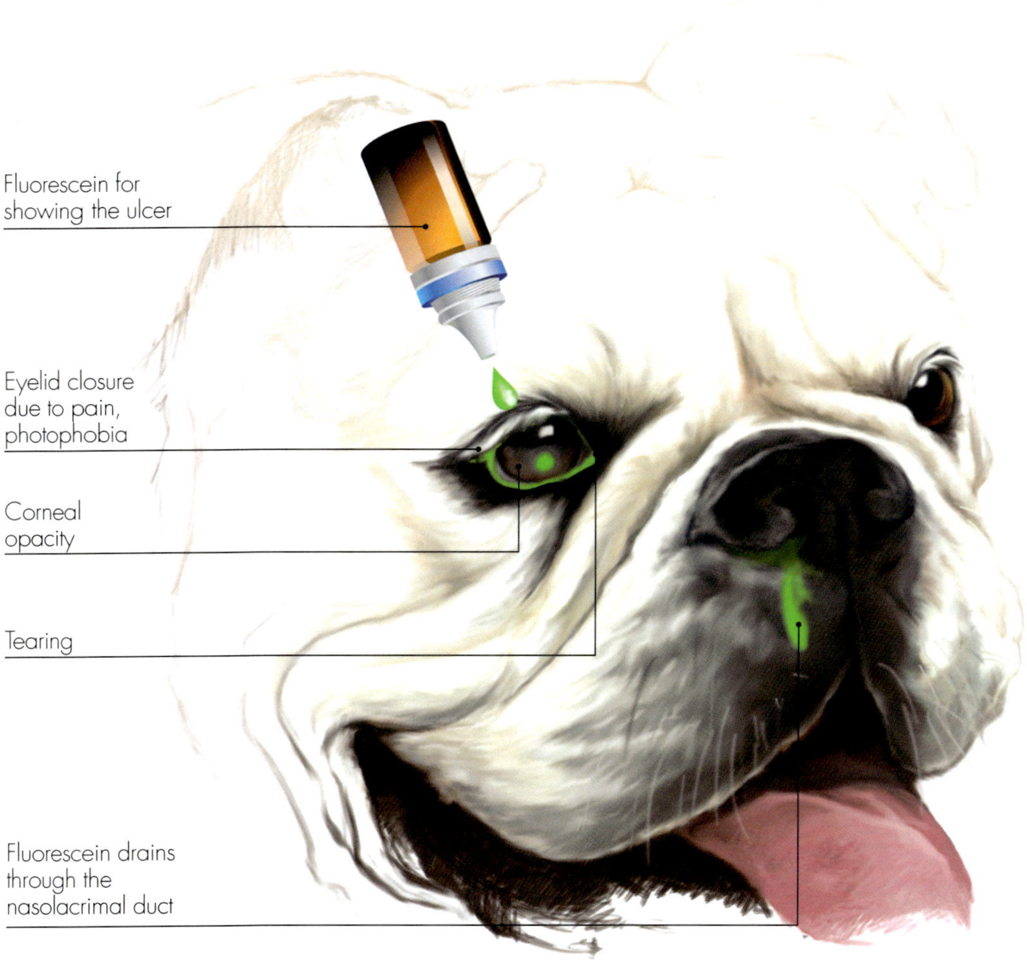

Damage to one or more layers of the cornea. They are classified into superficial and deep corneal ulcers, and descemetoceles.

Recurrent or indolent ulcers are refractory to medical treatment. The brachycephalic breeds (Boxer, Bulldog, Pug) are the most predisposed to this type.

Causes

- Trauma.
- Foreign bodies.
- Irritants.
- Continued hair rubbing.
- Keratoconjunctivitis sicca.
- Bacteria and viruses.

Pain and possible secondary infections must be tackled. Healing must be promoted.

Types of corneal ulcers

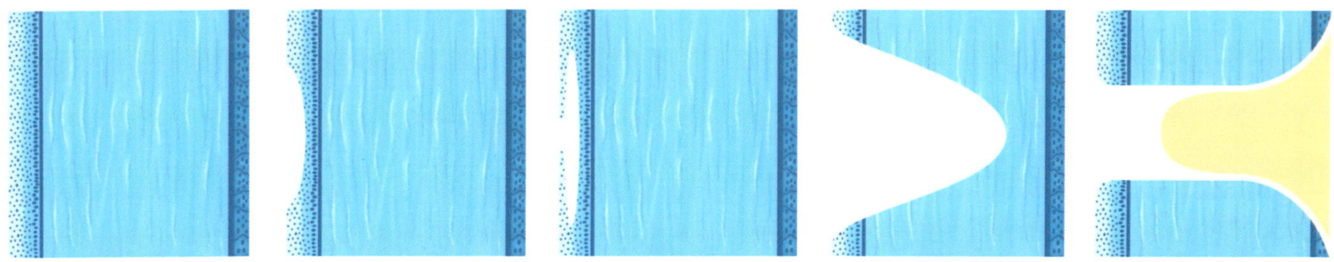

Surgical treatment

- Conjunctival flaps are applied in deep corneal lesions and descemetoceles. The flap fills the corneal defect, helps on its healing and avoid a corneal perforation.
- The defect can be covered stitching the third eyelid to the bulbar conjunctiva (tarsorrhaphy).
- Indolent and chronic ulcers must be carefully revived by scraping, milling techniques or grid keratectomies.

EYES

52 Degeneration of the lens

Cataracts

Cataracts are the partial or total loss of lens transparency. They can be uni- or bilateral and are classified according to their location, degree of maturation, age of onset and progression.

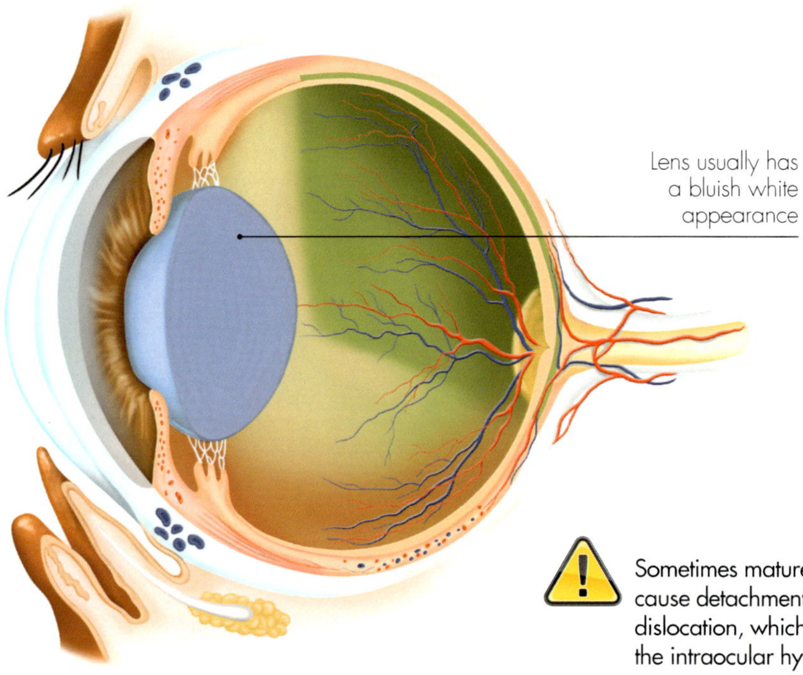

Sometimes mature cataracts cause detachment and lens dislocation, which stimulates the intraocular hypertension.

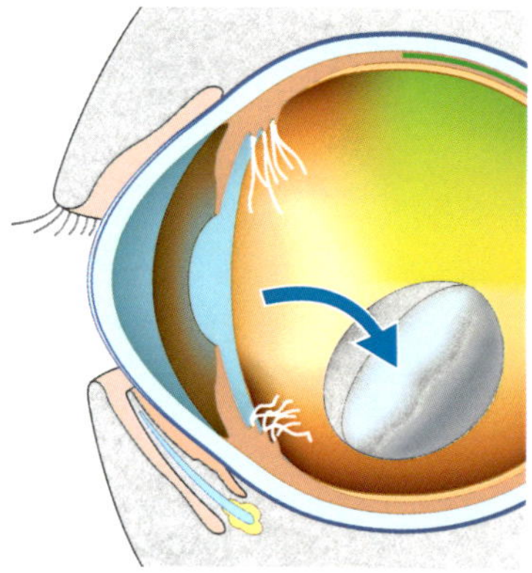

Posterior lens luxation (complete)

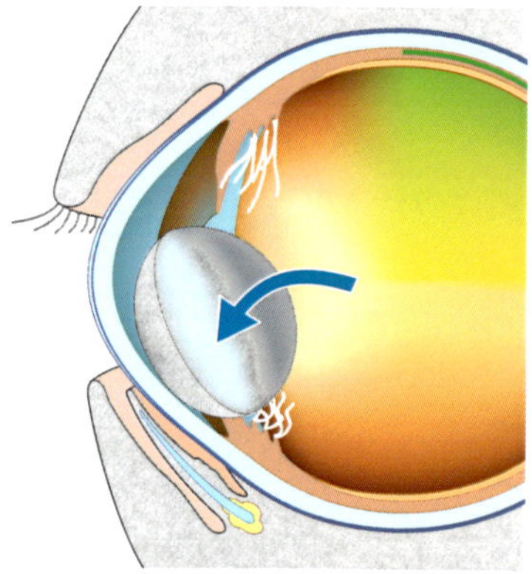

Anterior lens luxation

Causes

- Degenerative (frequently).
- Trauma.
- Metabolic disorders (diabetic cataract).
- Toxic.
- Genetic (congenital and juvenile cataract).
- Other eye conditions.

Surgical technique for the resolution of cataracts

Extracapsular extraction by phacoemulsification is the technique of choice. Ultrasounds are used to fragment lens, minimising risks, side effects and surgical time.

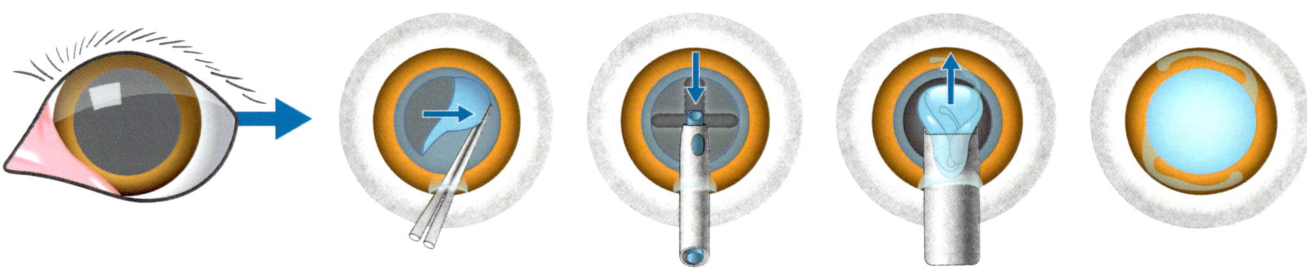

Small incision in the cornea | Rupture of the lens nucleus by ultrasound and extraction | Implantation of intraocular lens | The initial incision is closed without stitches

EYES

53 Eyelid and eyelash disorders

Eyelid disorders

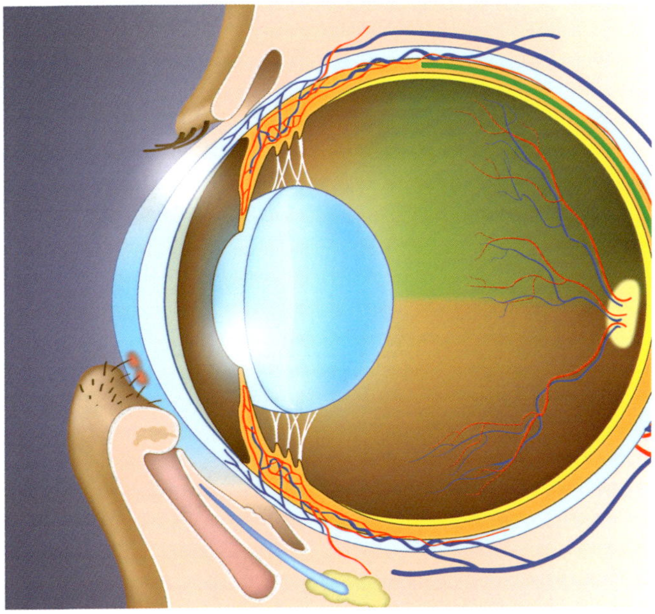

Entropion

Eyelid margin inversion which may be uni- or bilateral. It is noted:

- Excessive tearing, photophobia.
- Closed eyes by ocular discomfort.
- Keraritis and corneal ulcers by continuous hair rubbing.

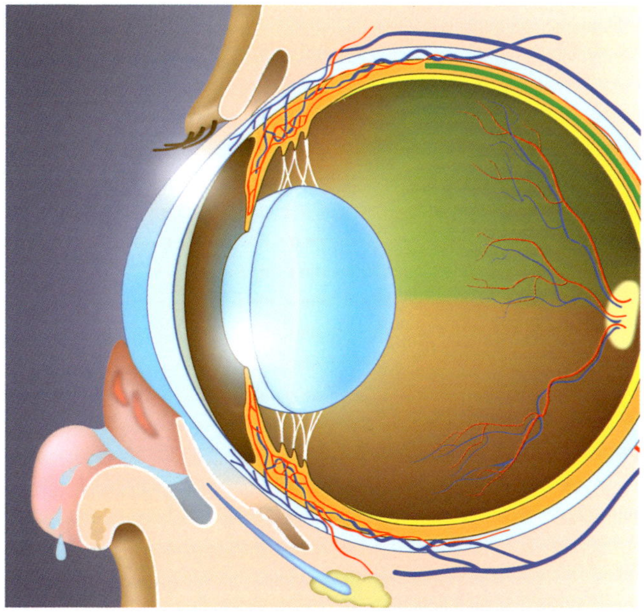

Ectropion

Eversion of the free edge of the eyelid, leaving the exposed conjunctiva and cornea unprotected. It is usually bilateral. It is noted:

- Conjunctival exposure.
- Excessive tearing.
- Chronic exposure keratitis.

Specialised surgery is required to solve these pathologies.

Eyelash disorders

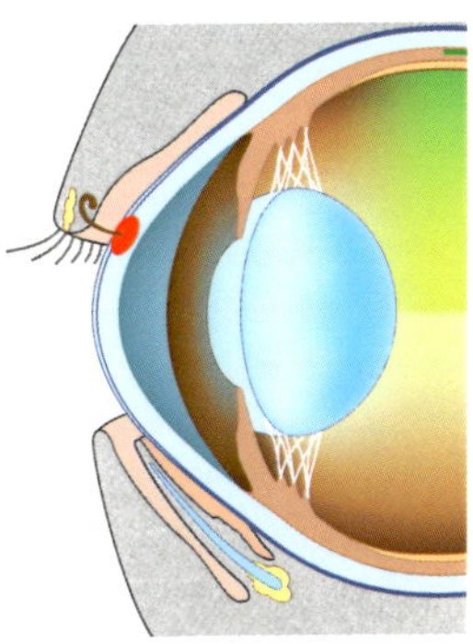

Ectopic cilia

Hairs in anomalous location grow from the conjunctiva and head towards the cornea.

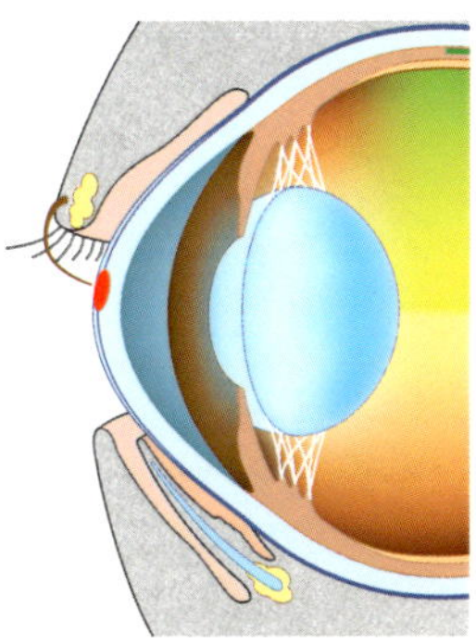

Trichiasis

Hairs in normal location headed towards the cornea. They are often associated with entropion.

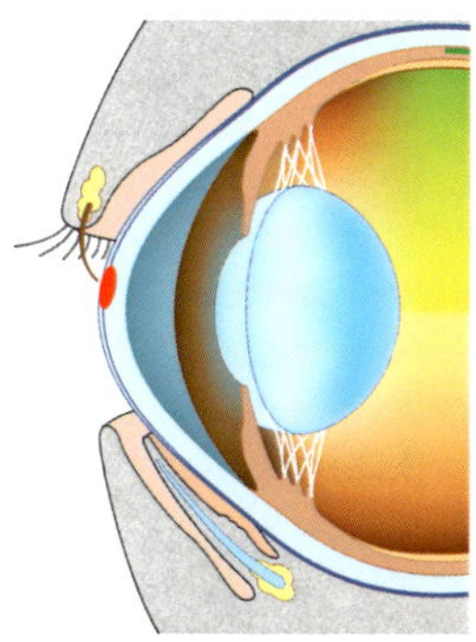

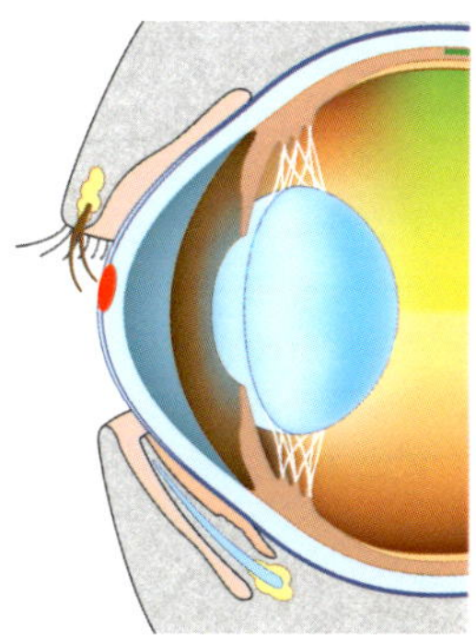

Distichiasis and districhiasis

Additional eyelashes in abnormal location may be headed towards the cornea. They usually emerge through secretion ducts of Meibomian glands of the upper eyelid. Districhiasis: if more than one hair goes through the same duct.

NERVOUS

54 Central, peripheral and autonomic nervous system

CENTRAL NERVOUS SYSTEM

A. Brain
B. Cerebellum
C. Brainstem
D. Spinal cord

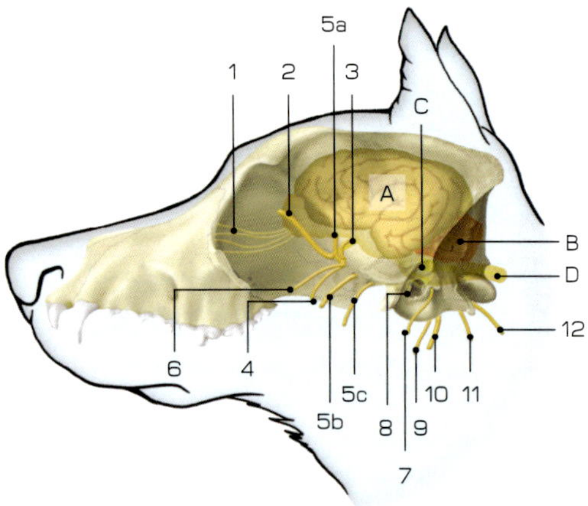

PERIPHERAL NERVOUS SYSTEM

1. Olfactory nerve (cranial nerve I)
2. Optic nerve (cranial nerve II)
3. Oculomotor nerve (cranial nerve III)
4. Trochlear nerve (cranial nerve IV)
5. Trigeminal nerve (cranial nerve V)
a. Ophthalmic branch (cranial nerve V1)
b. Maxillary branch (cranial nerve V2)
c. Mandibular branch (cranial nerve V3)
6. Abducens nerve (cranial nerve VI)
7. Facial nerve (cranial nerve VII)
8. Vestibulocochlear nerve (cranial nerve VIII)
9. Glossopharyngeal nerve (cranial nerve IX)
10. Vagus nerve (cranial nerve X)
11. Accessory nerve (cranial nerve XI)
12. Hypoglossal nerve (cranial nerve XII)
13. Cervical spinal nerves
14. Brachial plexus (C6, C7, C8 and T1)
15. Radial nerve
16. Musculocutaneous nerve
17. Median nerve
18. Ulnar nerve
19. Thoracic spinal nerves
20. Lumbar spinal nerves
21. Lumbosacral plexus (L3-L7 and S1-S3)
22. Femoral nerve
23. Saphenous nerve
24. Obturator nerve
25. Sciatic nerve
26. Cauda equina

AUTONOMIC NERVOUS SYSTEM

27. Cranial cervical ganglion
28. Distal vagal ganglion
29. Vagosympathetic trunk
30. Caudal cervical ganglion
31. Cervicothoracic ganglion
32. Vagus nerve
33. Vagus nerve, dorsal branch
34. Vagus nerve, ventral branch
35. Ganglia of the sympathetic trunk
36. Celiac-mesenteric ganglion
37. Caudal mesenteric ganglion
38. Hypogastric nerve

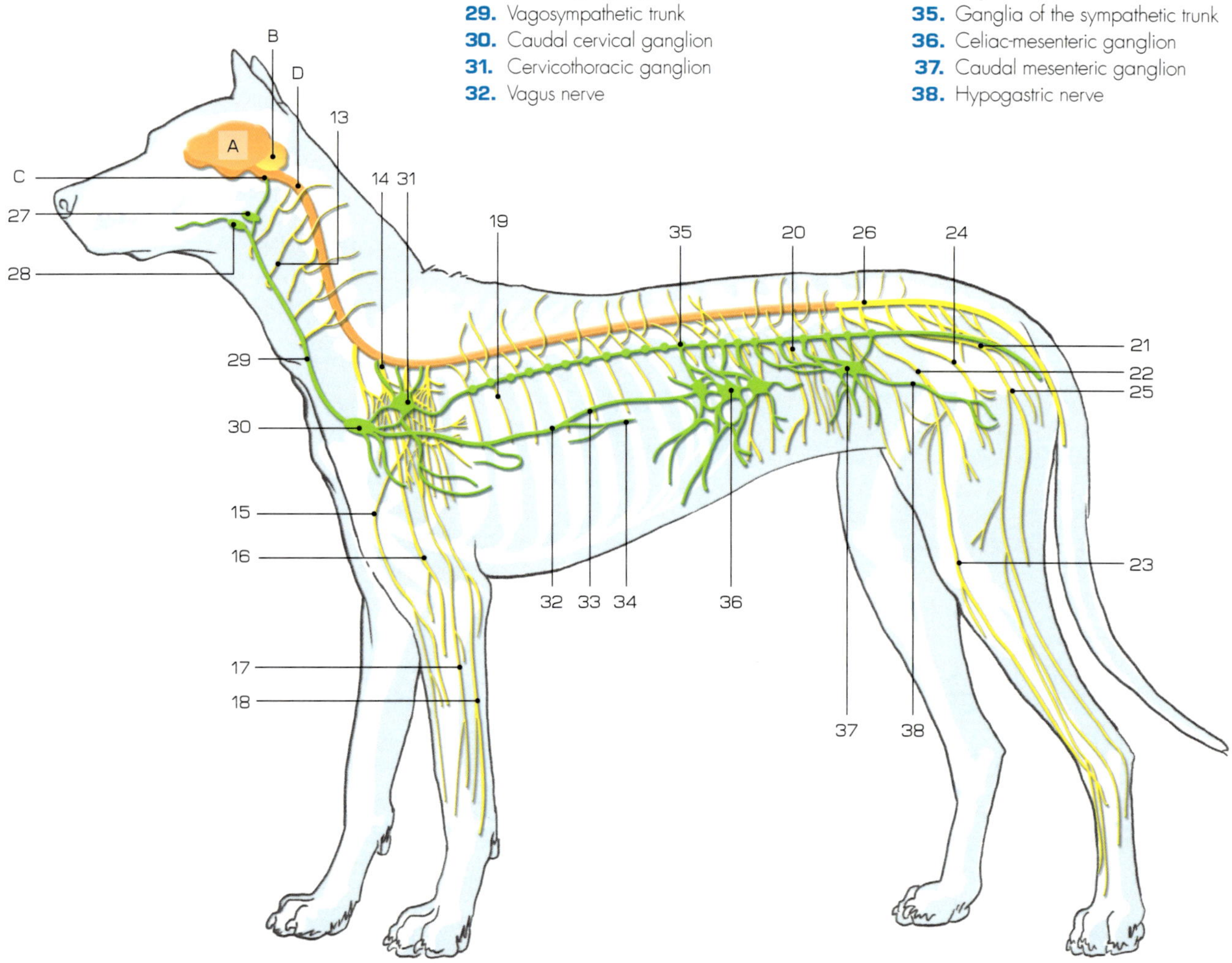

NERVOUS

55 Cognitive dysfunction syndrome (CDS)

Neurodegenerative disorder associated with age, which is manifested by behavioural changes. It can affect from 7 years of age, with an incidence of 33 % in dogs over 11 years.

Clinical signs

- Confusion and spatial and temporal disorientation.
- Changing relationships with family and other animals.
- Decreased activity.
- Irritability and anxiety, altered appetite.
- Low response to stimuli.
- Removal problems.
- Nocturnal activity, disturbed sleep / wakefulness.
- Lack of memory and learning.
- Emergence of compulsive behaviours.

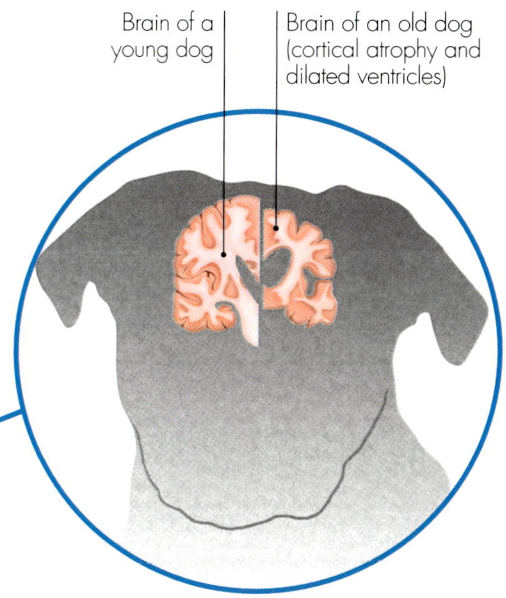

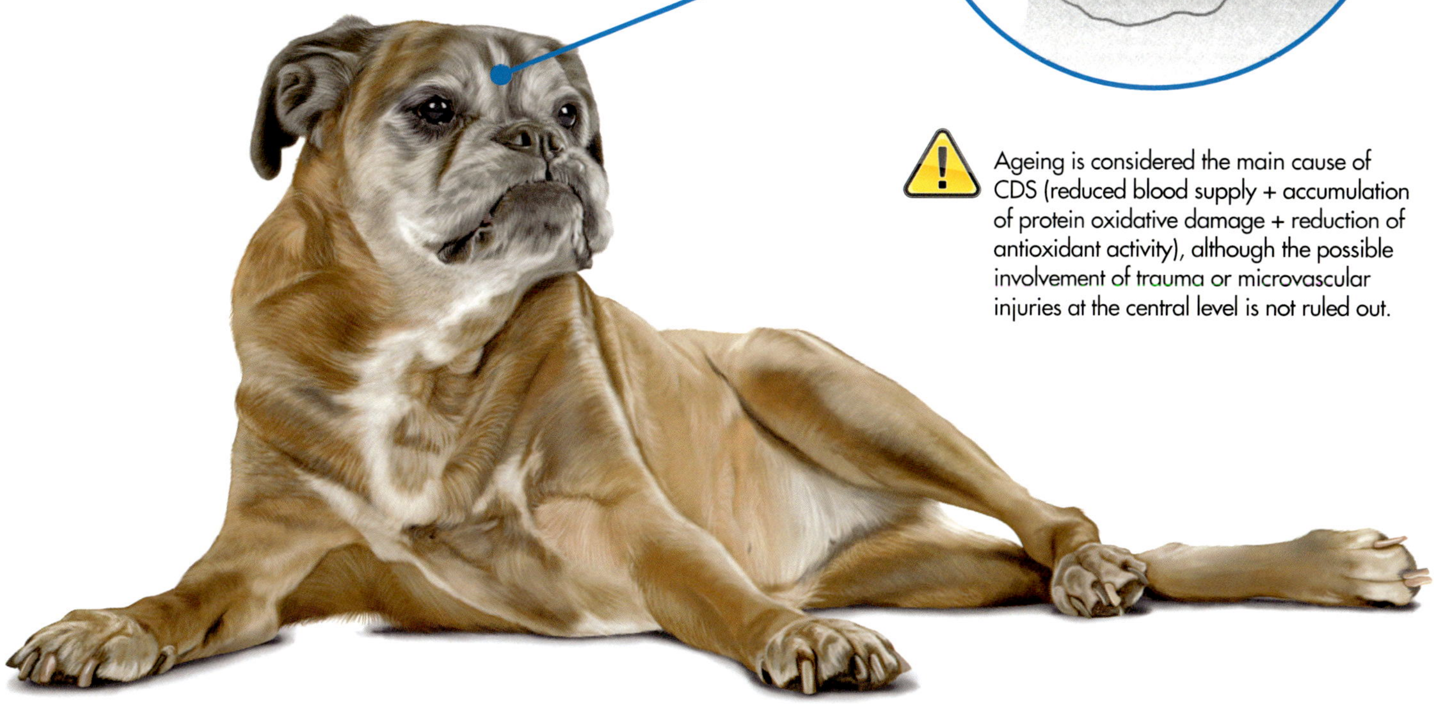

Ageing is considered the main cause of CDS (reduced blood supply + accumulation of protein oxidative damage + reduction of antioxidant activity), although the possible involvement of trauma or microvascular injuries at the central level is not ruled out.

Medical treatment

Drugs that improve cardiovascular performance and neurological function (neuroprotectives).

Dietary treatment

Supply of vitamins C and E, selenium, L-carnitine and triglycerides.

Recommendations

- Adapting the dog's environment to the new situation (go outdoors more frequently, leave some lights on at night).
- Apply stimulation programmes.
- Avoid a sedentary lifestyle.

NERVOUS

56 Peripheral and central vestibular syndrome

The vestibular system is located in the inner ear and in various areas of the central nervous system. Its dysfunction involves alterations in gait, posture of the head and movement of the eyeballs.

⚠ The idiopathic form, also called geriatric vestibular syndrome, occurs suddenly in aged animals.

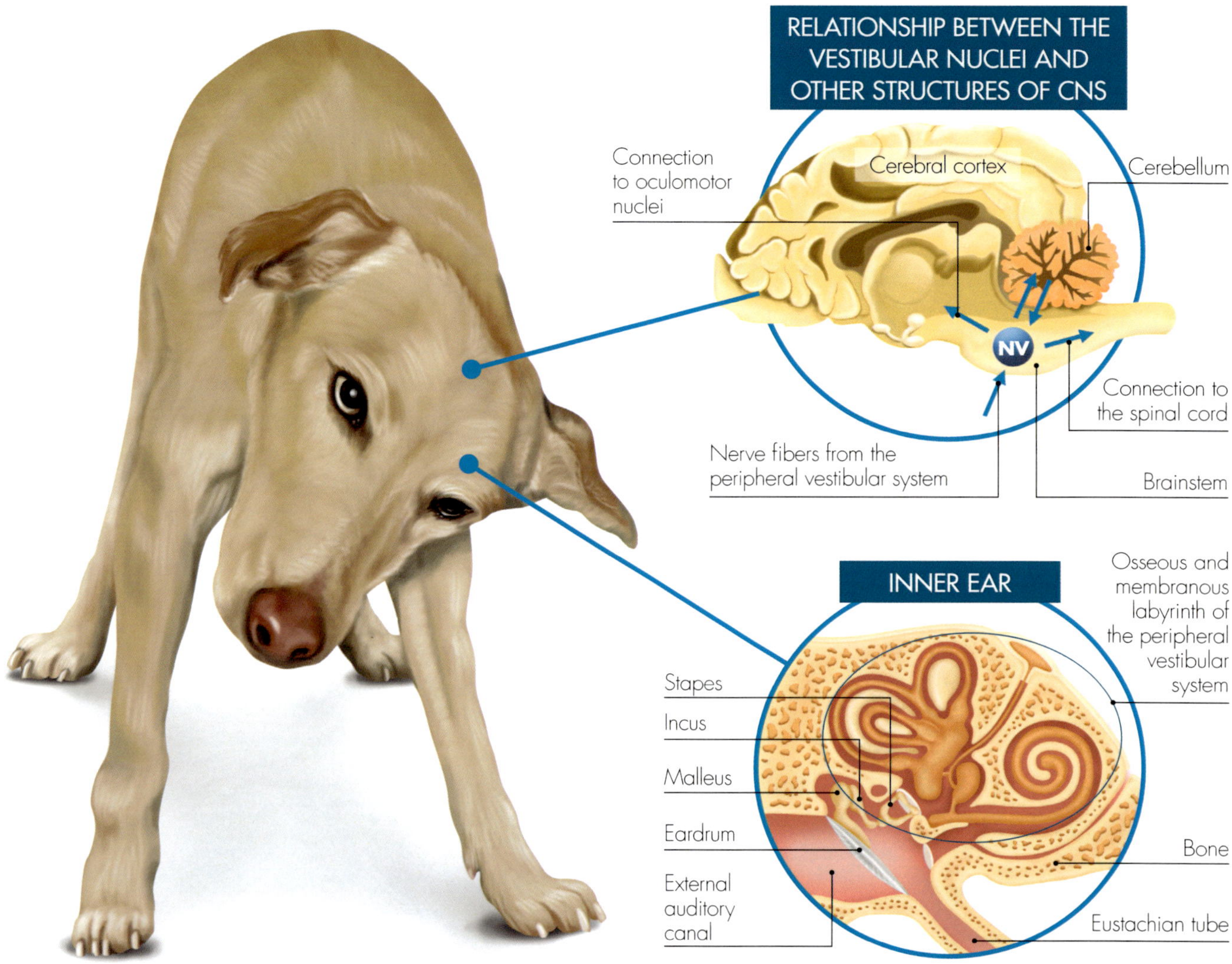

Causes

Peripheral vestibular syndrome

- Disorders in the middle and inner ear.
- Trauma.
- Idiopathic vestibular syndrome.
- Congenital malformations.
- Thyroid insufficiency.
- Drug toxicity.

Central vestibular syndrome

- Trauma.
- Cerebral haemorrhage.
- Encephalitis.
- Brain tumour.
- Drug toxicity.

Clinical signs

- Head tilt.
- Nystagmus: involuntary and rhythmic movement of the eyeballs.
- Vomiting due to dizziness.
- Positional strabismus.
- Vestibular ataxia: dogs tilt, fall or spin in circles.
- Possible Horner's syndrome.

57 Canine leishmaniasis

Mosquito disease

Parasitic disease caused by the protozoan *Leishmania infantum* and transmitted primarily through the bite of sandflies.

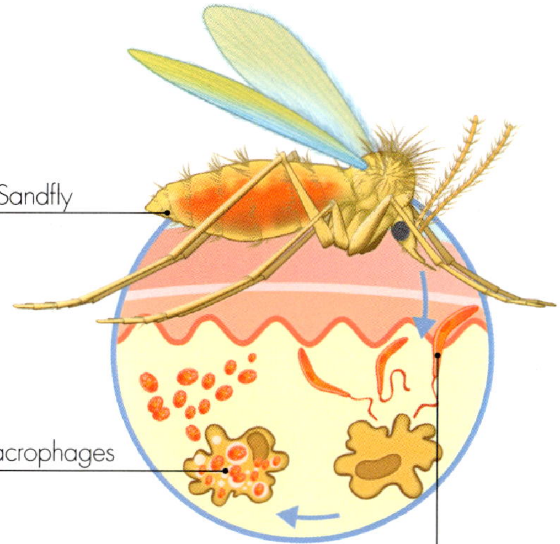

Worldwide distribution and endemic disease in the Mediterranean basin. It can be transmitted to humans (zoonosis).

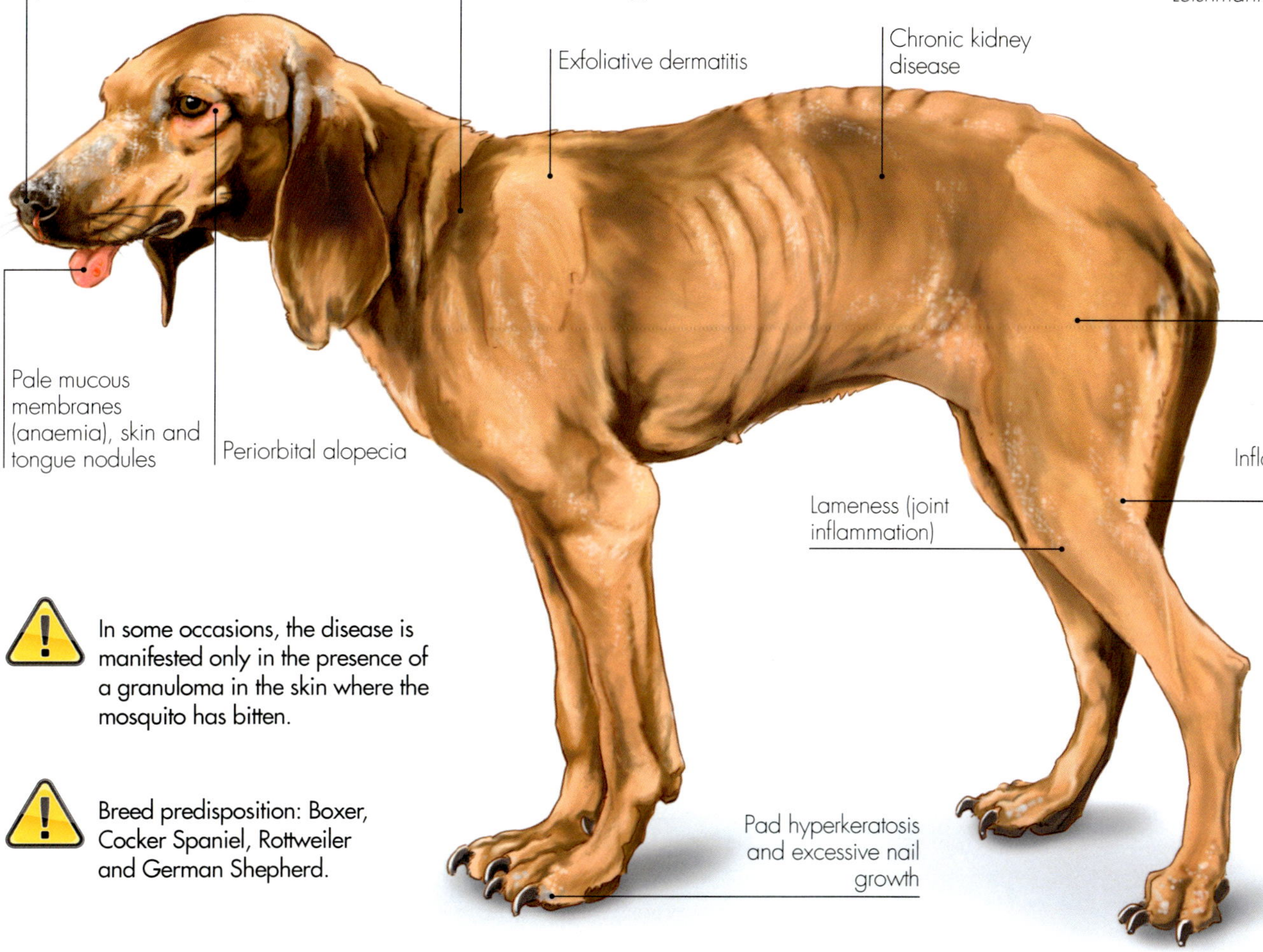

In some occasions, the disease is manifested only in the presence of a granuloma in the skin where the mosquito has bitten.

Breed predisposition: Boxer, Cocker Spaniel, Rottweiler and German Shepherd.

Medical treatment

- Combination of anti-leishmanial (pentavalent antimonials, miltefosine) and leishmaniostatic drugs (allopurinol).
- Complete parasite removal is not achieved, but symptoms are controlled.

Recommendations

- Repellents or topical insecticides (pipettes or collars) to prevent the bite of sandflies and, therefore, the transmission.
- Mosquito nets on doors and windows of the houses.
- Avoid late afternoon walks.
- Vaccination.

58 Filariasis

Heartworm disease

Disease caused by the parasite *Dirofilaria immitis* with worldwide distribution (areas of high temperature and moisture). It is transmitted by biting various species of mosquitoes that carry the parasite.

⚠ Chronic and severe course. Initially affects the pulmonary arteries, then the lung, and finally the heart.

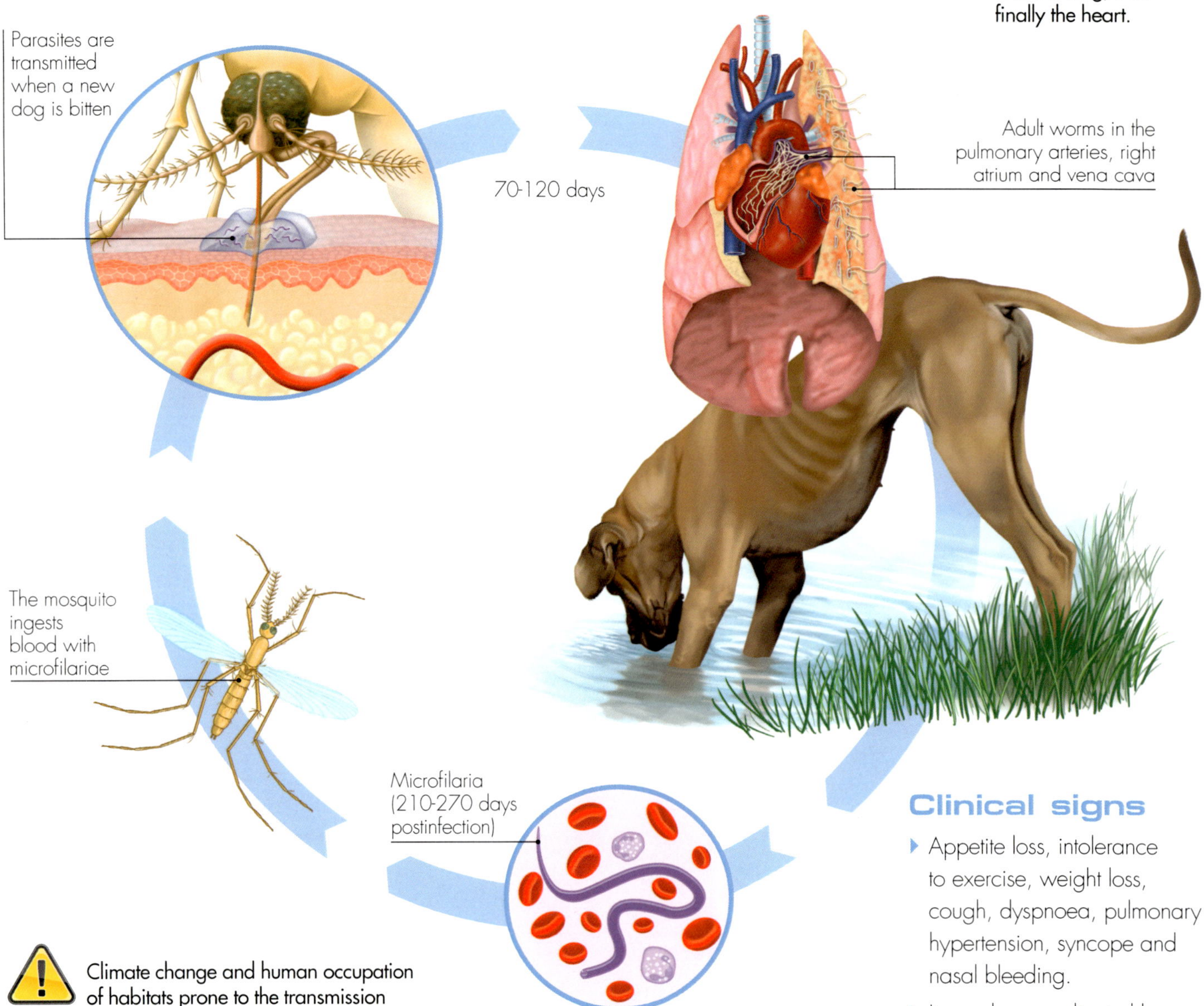

⚠ Climate change and human occupation of habitats prone to the transmission contribute to its spread.

Clinical signs

- Appetite loss, intolerance to exercise, weight loss, cough, dyspnoea, pulmonary hypertension, syncope and nasal bleeding.
- It may be complicated by ascites and oedema.

Medical treatment

Against adult heartworms and larvae, as well as to avoid parasitic thrombosis.

Surgical treatment

Heartworms can be removed by surgery in massive parasitoses.

Recommendations / prevention

- Continuous deworming.
- Annual assessment.
- Avoid mosquito bites (try not to go out at sunset in endemic areas).

59 Infectious diseases transmitted by ticks

Babesiosis, ehrlichiosis and Lyme disease

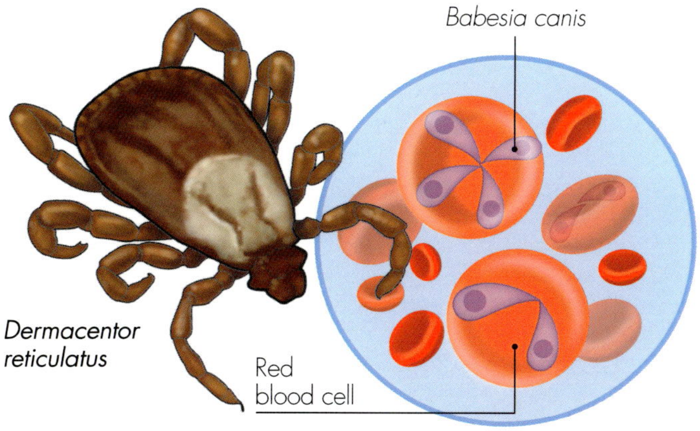

Babesiosis

Disease caused by protozoa of the genus *Babesia* and transmitted by ticks of different genus depending on the species of *Babesia* involved.

Clinical signs

- Hyperthermia.
- Haemolytic anaemia.
- Jaundice.
- Haemoglobinuria.
- Lethargy.
- Anorexia.

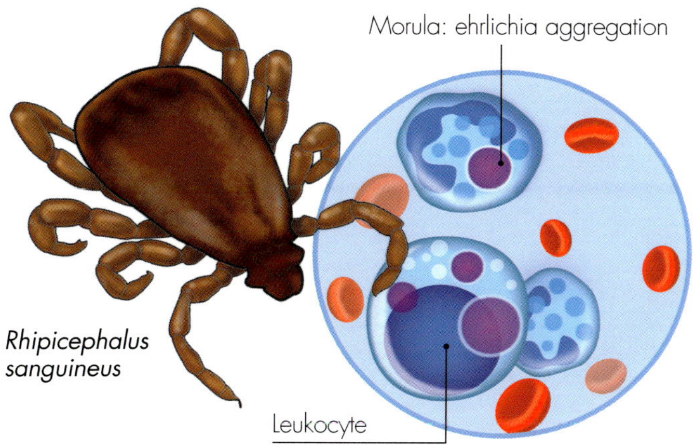

Ehrlichiosis

Disease caused by the bacterium *Ehrlichia canis* and transmitted by the tick *Rhipicephalus sanguineus*.

Clinical signs

- Depression, fever, lymphadenopathy, splenomegaly, vomiting, lameness, dyspnoea, weight loss.
- Prone to bleeding (skin and nose).
- Ocular: uveitis, hyphaema, retinal detachment and blindness.
- In chronic phase, joint, kidney and neurological signs appear.

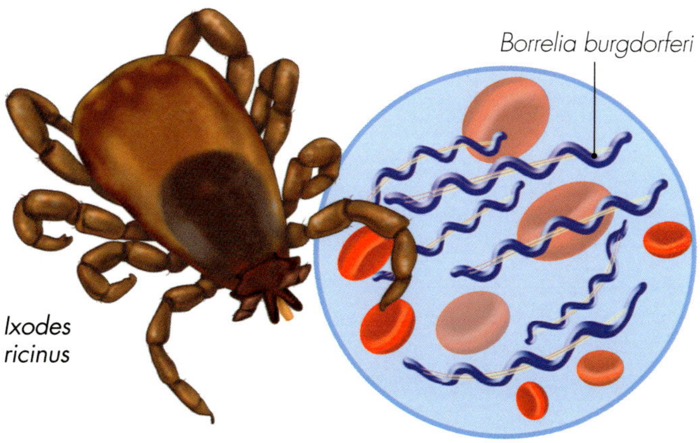

Lyme disease

Disease caused by the bacterium *Borrelia burgdorferi* and transmitted by ticks of the genus *Ixodes*.

Clinical signs

- Recurrent limb lameness (arthritis).
- Glomerulonephritis.
- Vomiting, diarrhoea, anorexia, weight loss, polyuria / polydipsia, ascites and oedema.

Recommendations / prevention

- Control of ticks: baths, sprays, pyrethroid collars and pipettes, amitraz, fipronil and imidacloprid.
- Avoid tick-infested areas.

Disease transmissible to humans (zoonosis).

60 Canine parvovirus

Disease caused by a *Parvovirus*. It is the most frequent cause of viral enteritis in puppies (6 weeks-6 months). It is more severe in puppies with rapid growth and usually occurs in spring and summer. It is primarily transmitted orally.

Parvovirus is resistant in the environment for months. It is inactivated only with diluted bleach solution (1 part in 27 of water).

More sensitive breeds

- Rottweiler.
- Doberman.
- Labrador Retriever.
- American Pitbull Terrier.
- German Shepherd.
- Yorkshire Terrier.

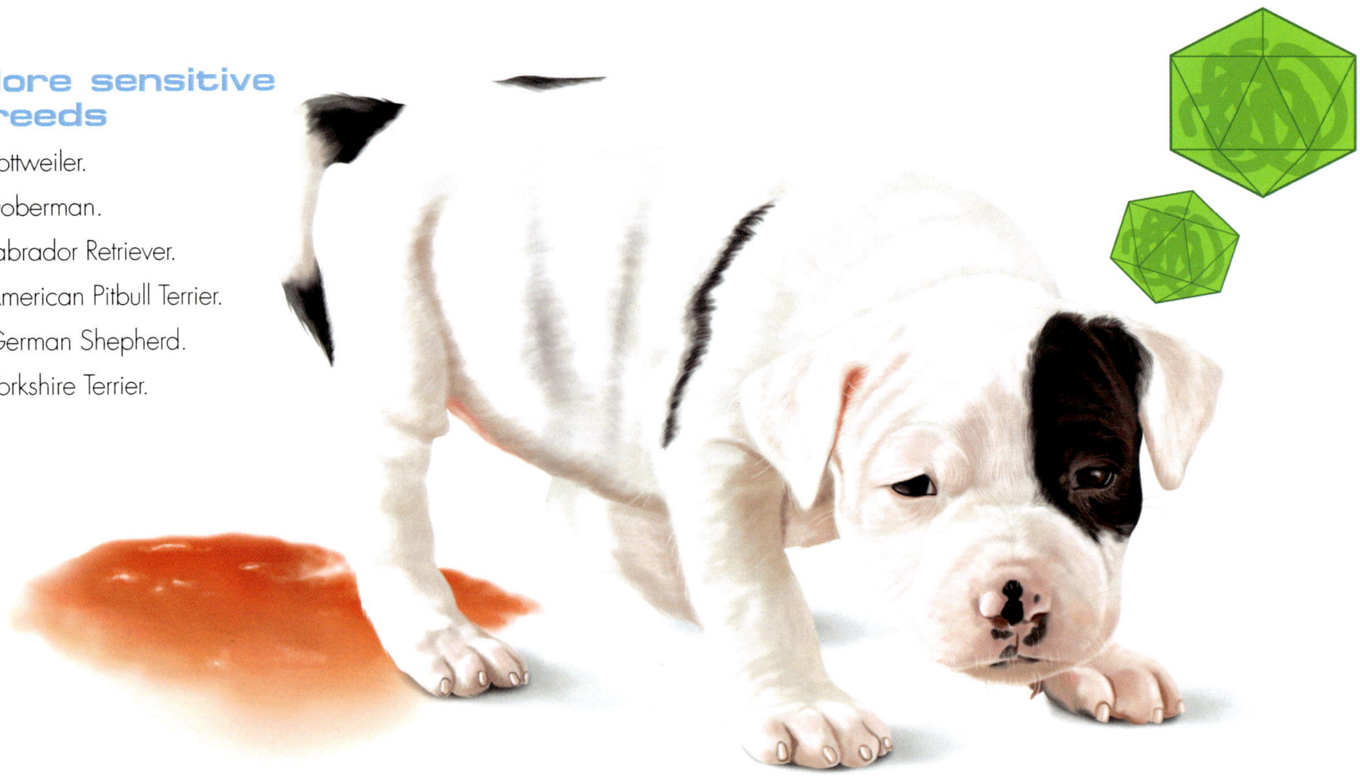

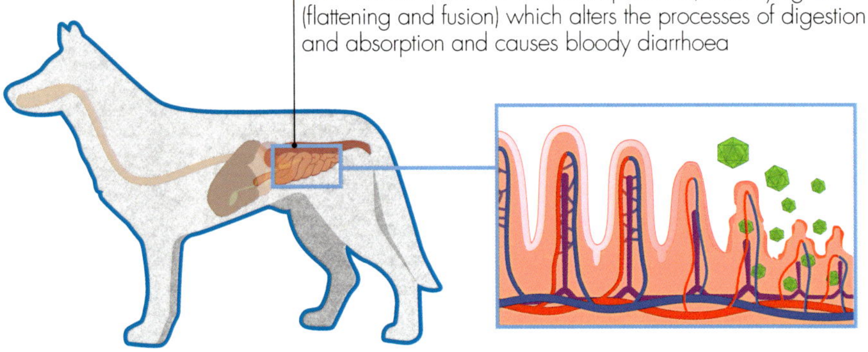

The virus colonises the intestinal epithelium, destroying villi (flattening and fusion) which alters the processes of digestion and absorption and causes bloody diarrhoea

Clinical signs

Cardiac form (intrauterine or perinatal infection)

- Puppies <8 weeks old.
- They can die from acute myocardial infection (myocarditis).
- Those who overcome myocarditis may subsequently die from congestive heart failure.

Enteric form

- Fever, vomiting and diarrhoea: dehydration.
- Sepsis, hypovolaemic or septic shock.
- Death associated with severe dehydration conditions.

Medical treatment

Intense fluidotherapy, and vomiting and secondary bacterial infections control.

Secondary bacterial infections are crucial in the development of the clinical picture.

61 Canine distemper

Highly contagious disease caused by a *Morbillivirus*, whose severity depends largely on the immune response of the host. The virus is spread through secretions from the respiratory and digestive system, and also in the urine.

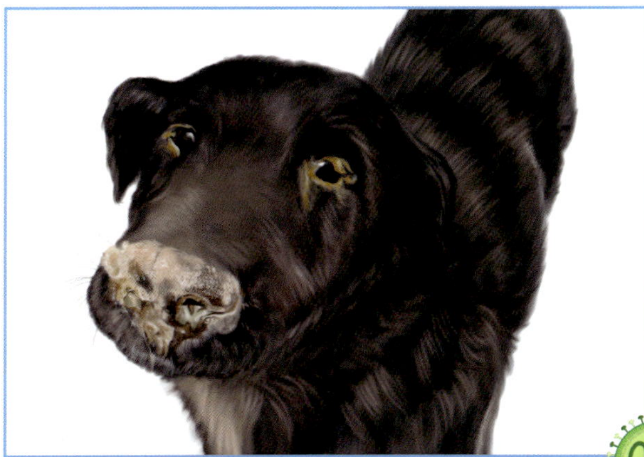

1º. Mucopurulent nasal discharge and conjunctivitis

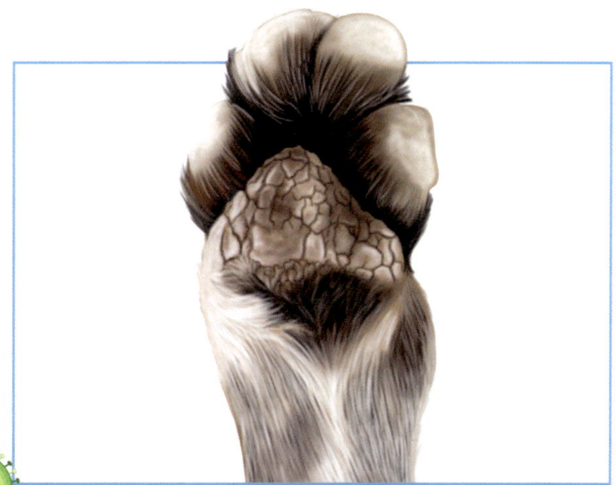

2º. Pad and muzzle hyperkeratosis

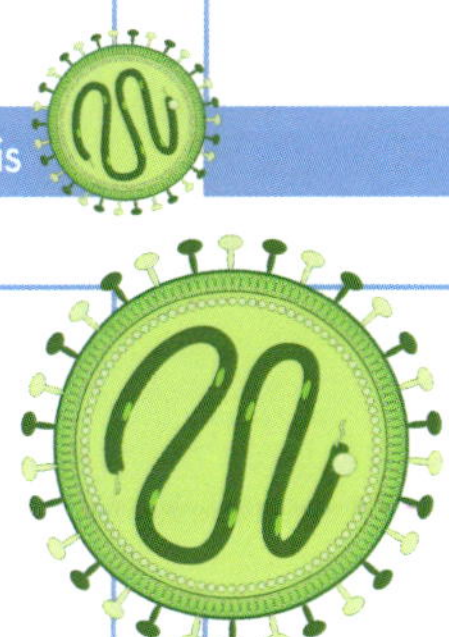

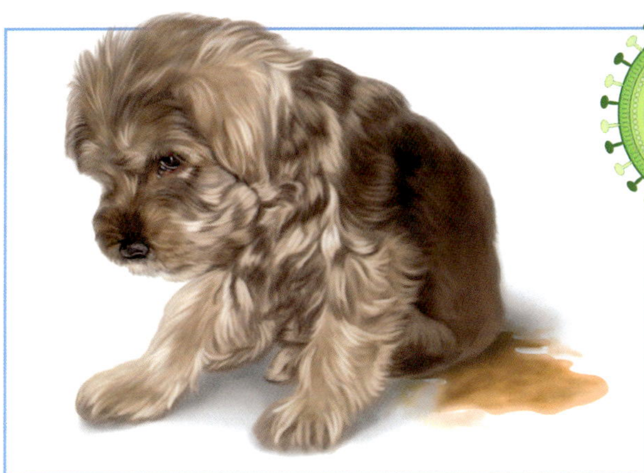

3º. Diarrhoea and dehydration

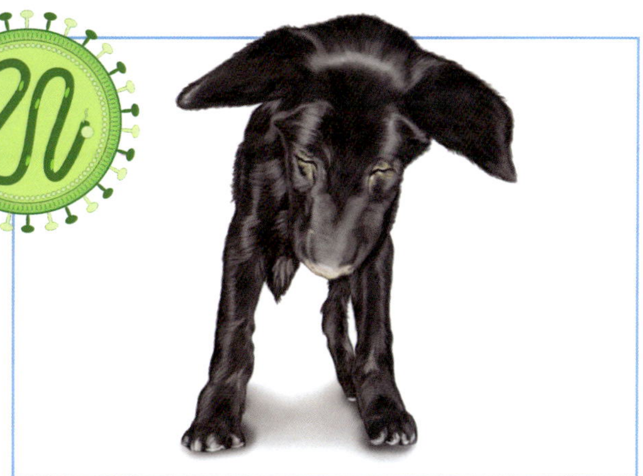

4º. Nervous symptoms

Acute form

- General symptoms (fever).
- Oculonasal: mucus, conjunctivitis, keratitis and corneal ulcers.
- Skin: pyodermatitis, hyperkeratosis (muzzle and footpads).
- Respiratory: cough, breath sounds and dyspnoea.
- Digestive: diarrhoea, isolated vomiting, dehydration and anorexia. Dental enamel hypoplasia.
- Nervous: neck stiffness, hyperesthaesia, ataxia, myoclonus, convulsions, paresis, etc.

Chronic form

- Progressive nervous signs.

Medical treatment

- There is no specific treatment. It is aimed at relieving symptoms.
- Prevent infection by vaccination (the best option).

Unvaccinated puppies of 3-6 months of age are the most prone to infection due to decreasing of maternal immunity.

62 Leptospirosis

Bacterial disease caused by pathogenic species of the genus *Leptospira*, which presents with acute kidney and liver infection and sometimes septicaemia. It is more common in large breed dogs living in contact with nature. Placenta and foetus are affected in pregnant females.

Zoonosis transmitted from the urine of infected animals, mainly rats, which infects water.

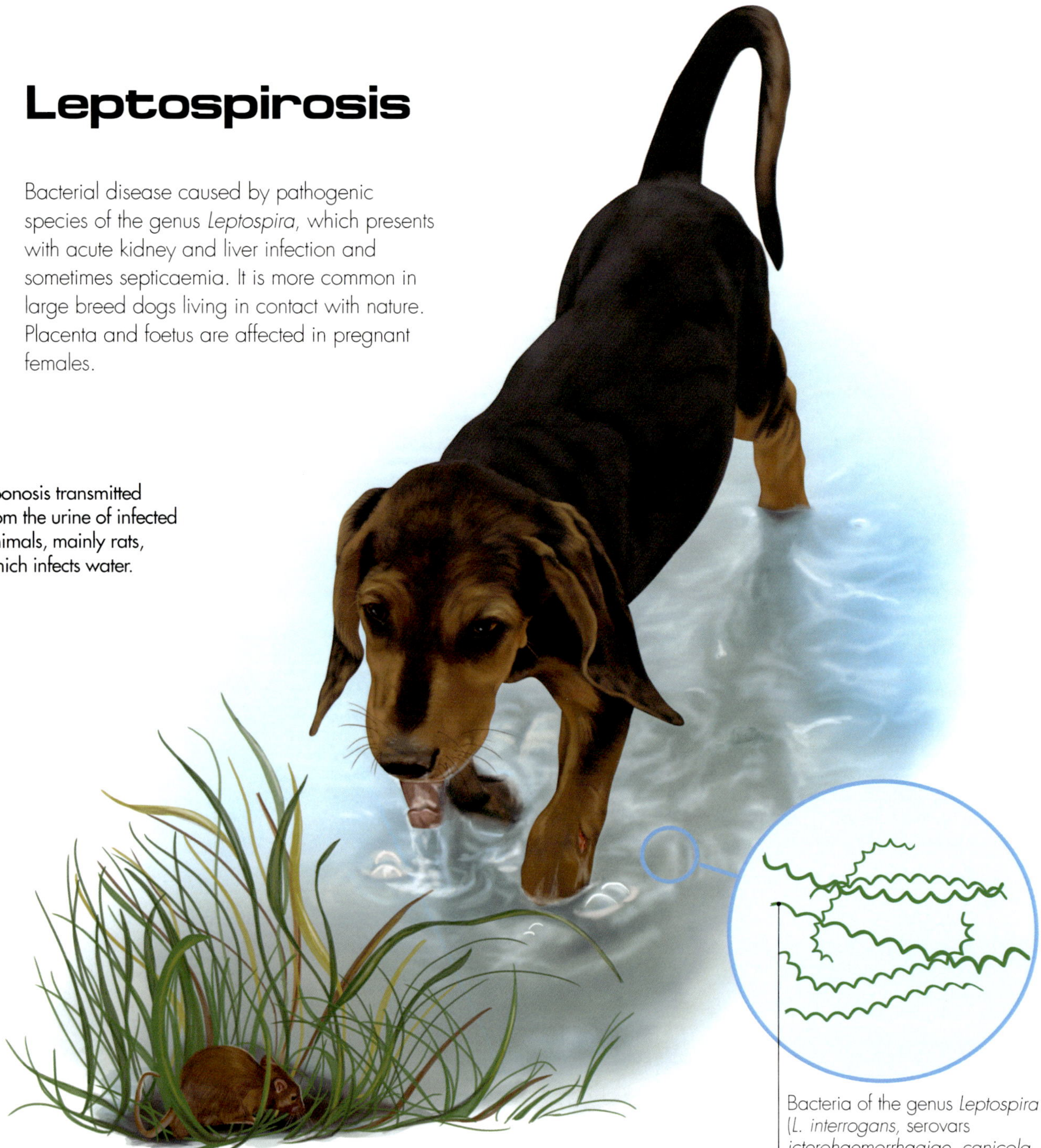

Bacteria of the genus *Leptospira* (*L. interrogans*, serovars *icterohaemorrhagiae*, *canicola* and *pomona*)

Infection can be orally or through skin wounds.

Medical treatment

Antibiotics and supportive therapy against clinical signs (hydration, recovery of renal function, liver protectors, etc.).

Clinical signs

- Depend on the age and immunity of the host, environmental factors and virulence of the infecting bacteria.
- They range from almost non-existent to deadly, and are presented in a hyperacute, acute or chronic form.
- Classical form:
  - High fever, lethargy, mucous congestion, conjunctivitis.
  - Abdominal pain, vomiting and diarrhoea.
  - Jaundice, hepatomegaly.
  - Severe renal impairment that can leave permanent damage in the kidney.
  - Neuromuscular pain and meningitis.

63 Kennel cough

Infectious tracheobronchitis

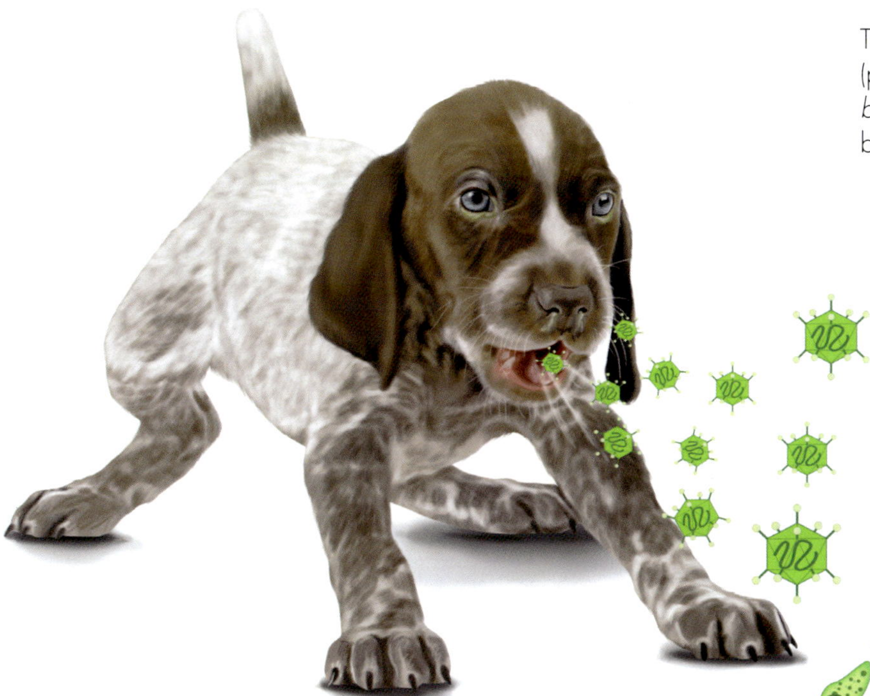

Tracheobronchial condition in which viral (parainfluenza), bacterial (*Bordetella bronchiseptica*) and mycoplasma agents may be involved, alone or in combination.

Highly contagious disease transmitted by inhalation.

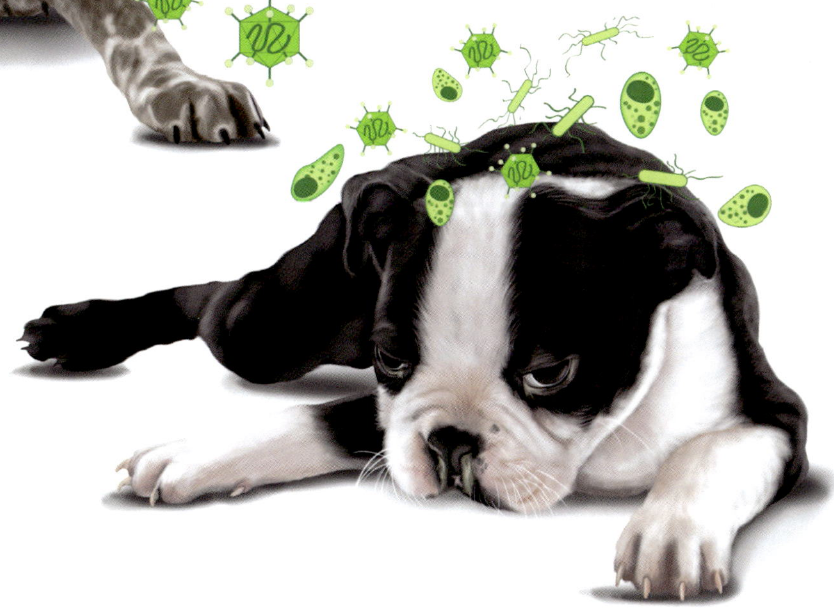

The clinical picture is more severe with the joint participation of several infectious agents.

Predisposing factors

- Unvaccinated animals.
- Communities.
- Young age (most severe).
- High prevalence in greyhounds and small and toy breeds (brachycephalic).
- Congenital disorders of the respiratory tree or chronic bronchitis.
- Cold months.

Clinical signs

Mild form (an infectious agent)

- Paroxysmal cough, mucopurulent rhinitis and conjunctivitis.
- Nausea and foamy respiratory secretions.

Severe form (several infectious agents)

- Fever, lethargy, dyspnoea, anorexia, mucopurulent discharge, weight loss.
- Chronic bronchitis as aftermath.
- The youngest and weakest may die.

Medical treatment

- Antibiotics and bronchodilators.
- Aerosol therapy using nebulisers.

Recommendations / prevention

- Appropriate vaccination program.
- Avoid prolonged exposure to cold.
- Avoid contact and sharing feeder with symptomatic dogs.

64 Rabies

Fatal disease caused by a virus of the *Rhabdoviridae* family, genus *Lyssavirus*, which affects the central nervous system of domestic and wild animals. It is present on all continents except Antarctica and is notifiable.

Global impact

- Kills 70,000 people in the world each year: the main victims are children in developing countries. Africa and Asia are the most affected areas.
- The dog is the main vector of rabies in these countries.

It is transmitted to humans through contact with infected saliva via bites or scratches.

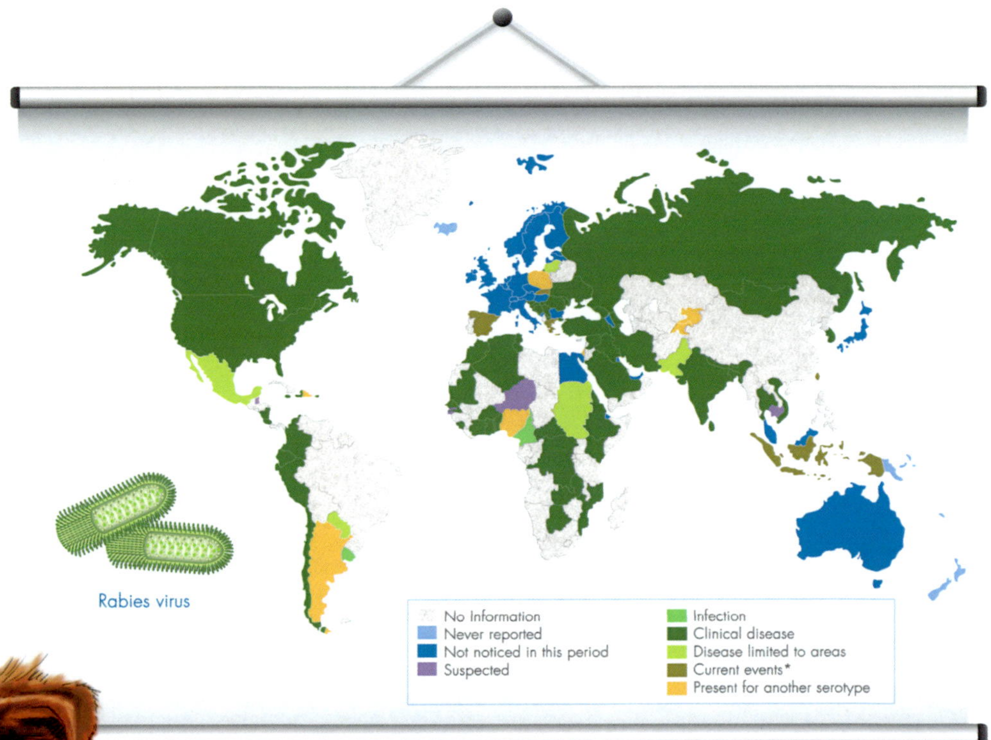

* Domestic rabies case in course in Spain during the first half of 2013 was resolved during the second one. There is a current event in France on February 2014.

This map is based on data provided by OIE (January-July 2013) for domestic and wildlife rabies of unspecified serotype.

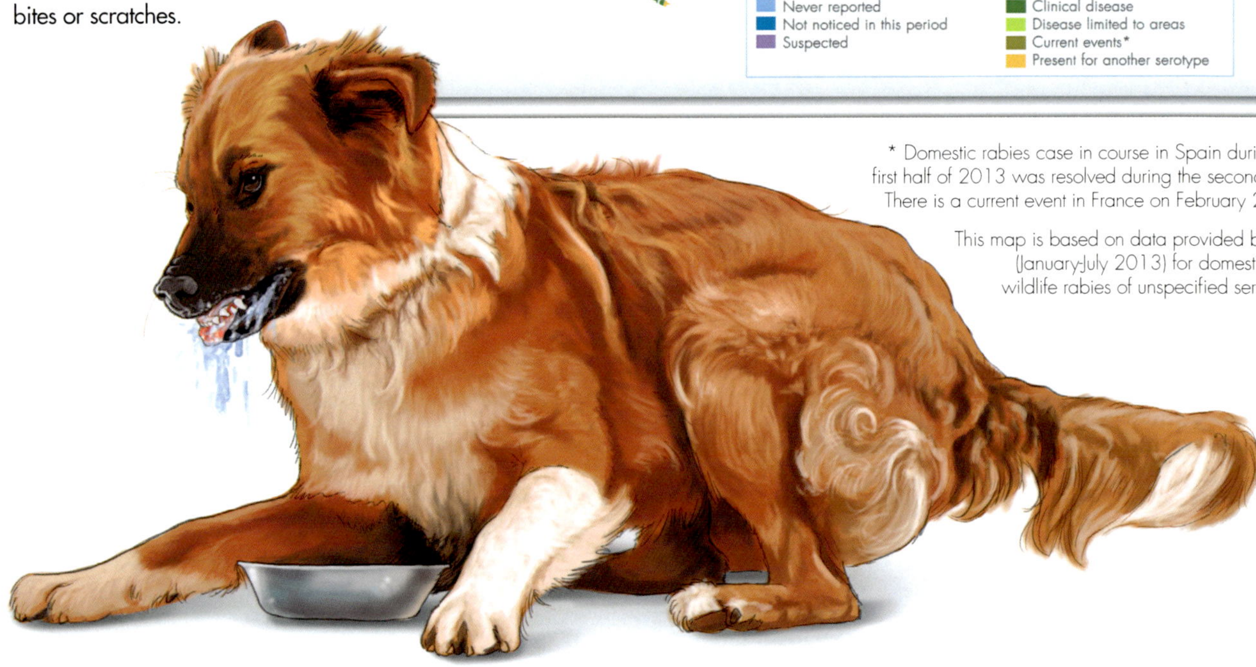

Clinical signs

- Receive a bite weeks ago.
- Sudden changes in behaviour (irritable, aggressive).
- Severe agitation alternating with depression.
- Characteristic bark (loud and furious), paralysis of masticatory muscles (hydrophobia, inability to eat, drooling).
- Progressive paralysis resulting in death.

Recommendations / prevention

- Vaccination programmes in companion animals (depend on each autonomous community), and vaccination and control of stray animals.
- Remove or reduce the disease in foxes by baiting with live vaccines.

65 Nail trimming

The excessive length of the nails can lead to snag somewhere and pull up, dig into the surrounding tissues and even a bad finger support that hinders the dog's gait or cause deformity in the fingers.

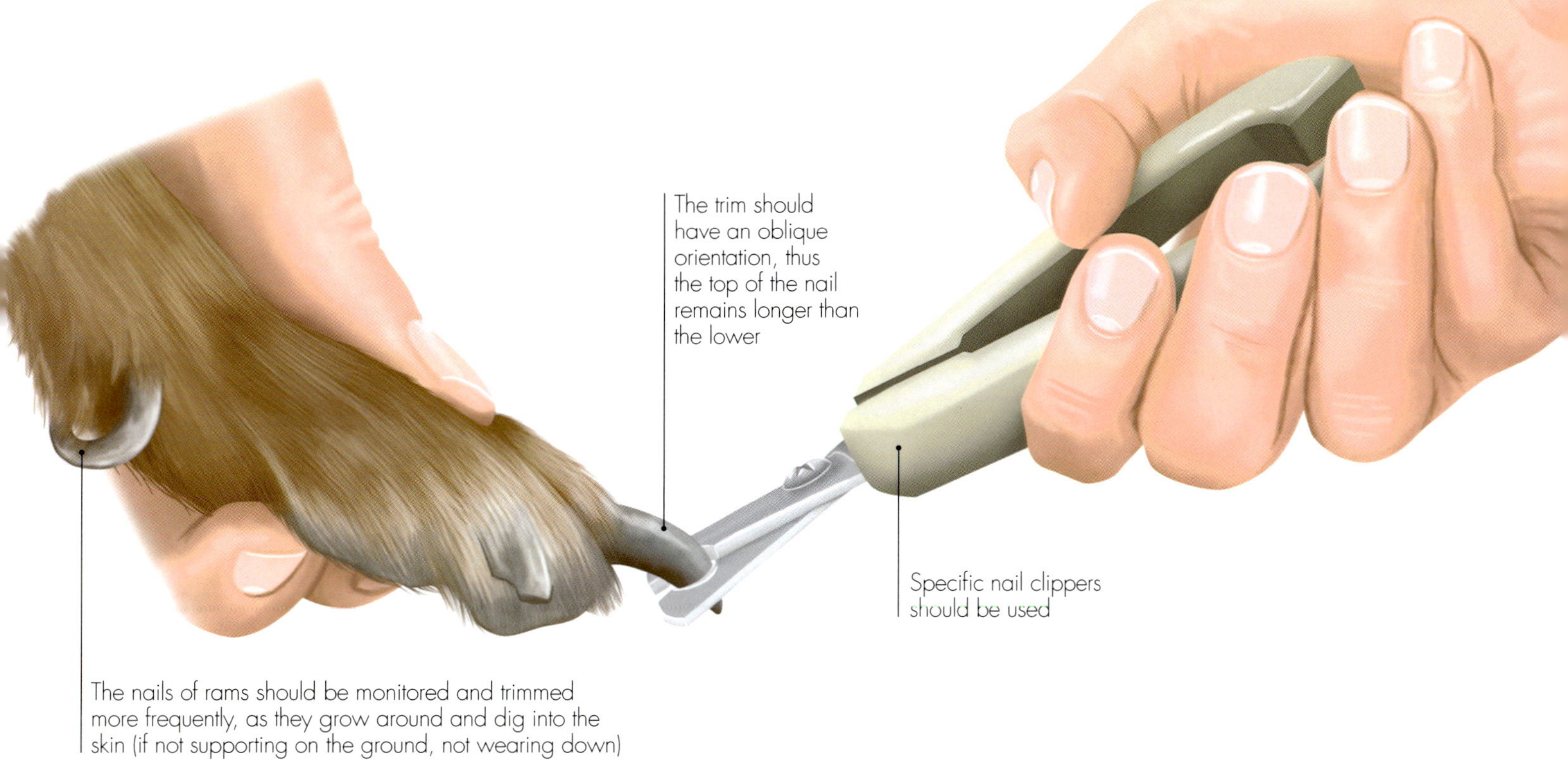
The trim should have an oblique orientation, thus the top of the nail remains longer than the lower
Specific nail clippers should be used
The nails of rams should be monitored and trimmed more frequently, as they grow around and dig into the skin (if not supporting on the ground, not wearing down)

If the nails are too long, it is better to go slowly trimming them to allow the retraction of the arteriovenous endings.

Dogs should be accustomed from puppies to be able to manipulate their paws and nails, thus this procedure will be more acceptable to them.

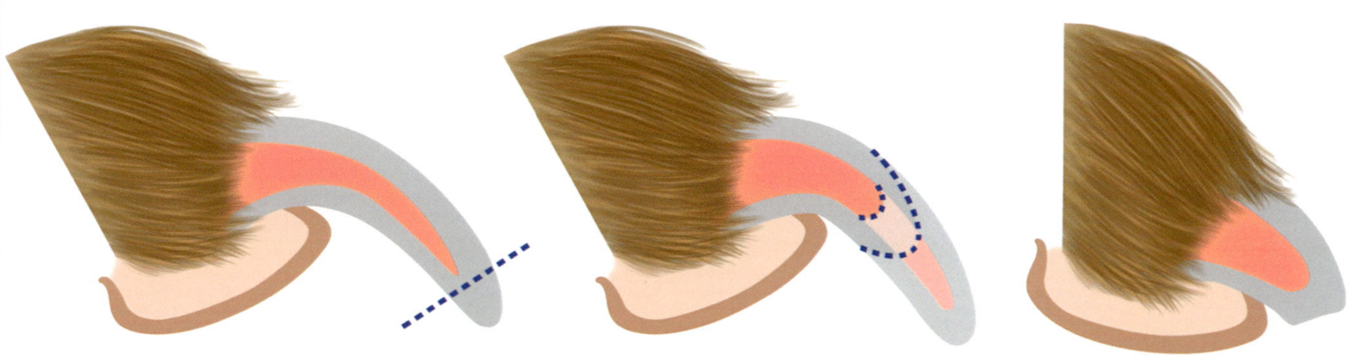

The nail root, with its nerve endings and blood vessels, will grow as nails grow.

Trimming a dog's nails regularly will lead to the quick retracting back over time.

Optimal appearance of the nail.

66 Problems caused by grass awns

Removal by means of crocodile forceps

Auditory canal

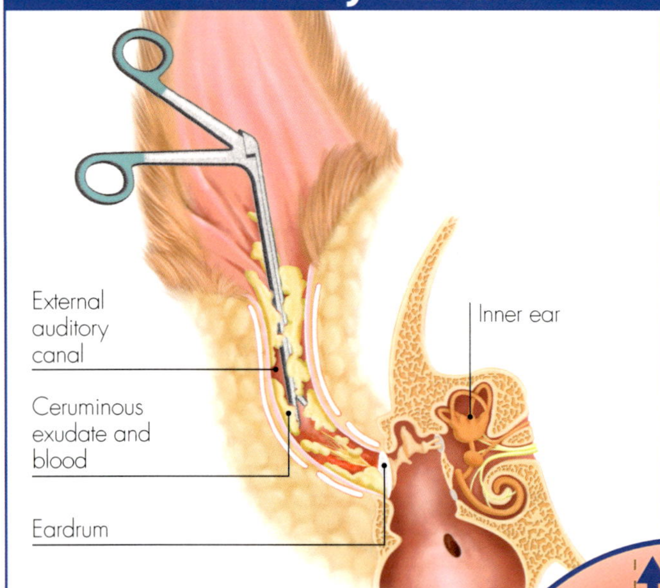

Interdigital space

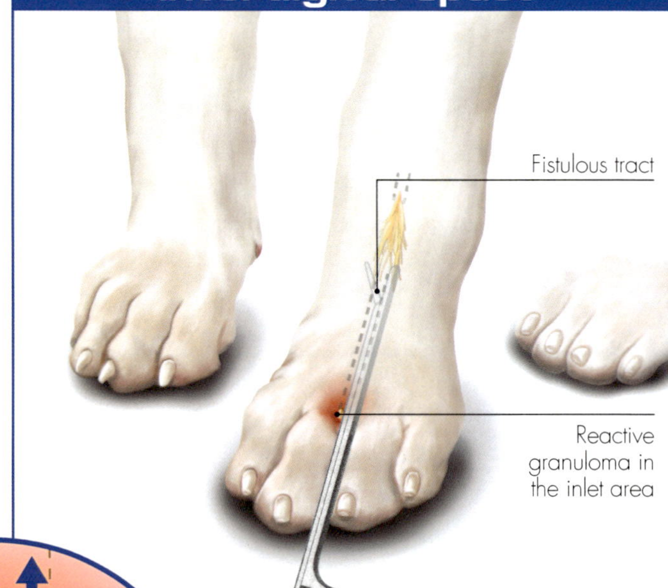

If grass awn has deepened a lot in the nasal turbinates, endoscopic techniques should be used for its removal.

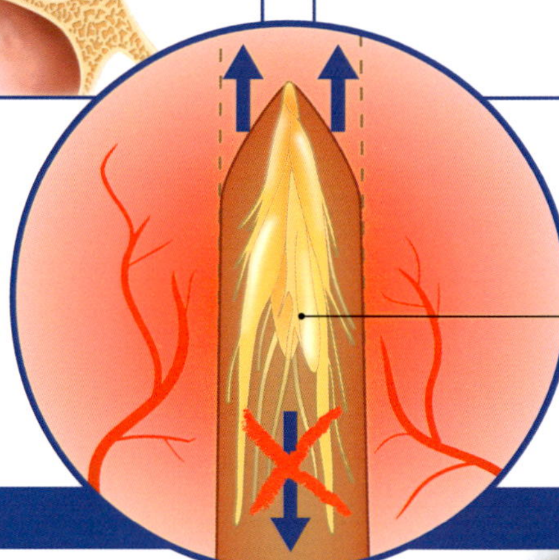

Nose

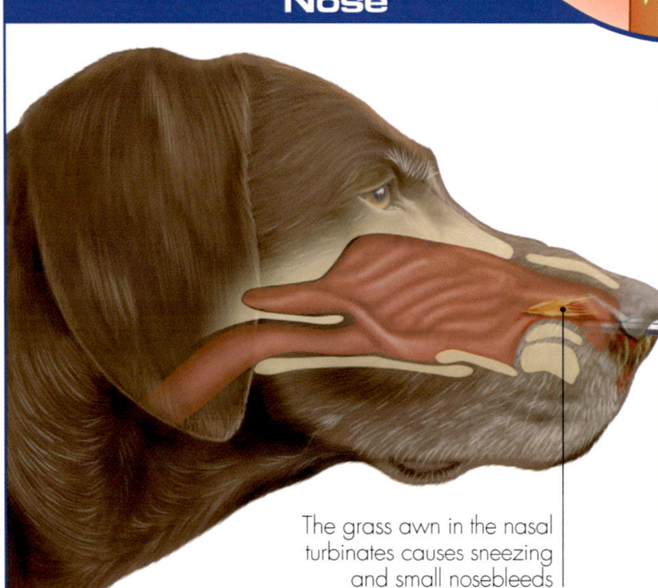

Eye

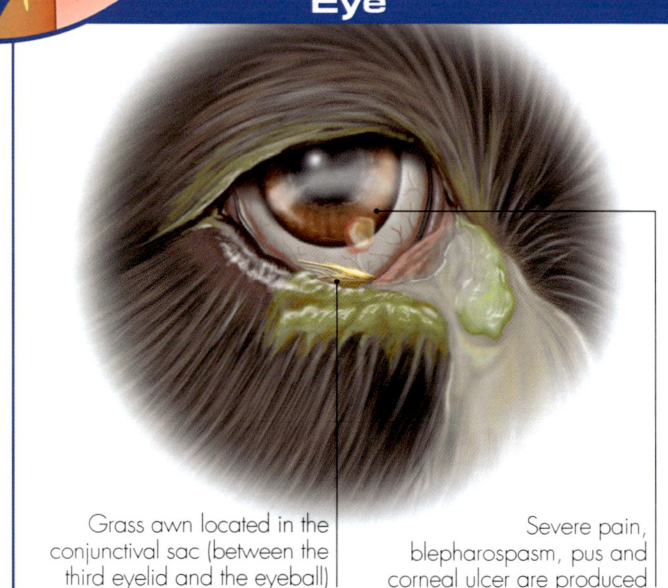

67 How to administer drugs

Orally

Tablets

The tablet must be placed as deeply as possible on the tongue (swallowing reflex)

When its mouth is opened, the upper lips must be pushed inwards

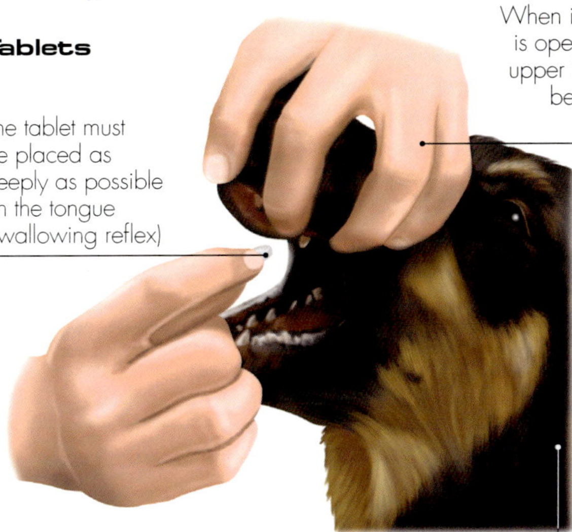

Head up diagonally

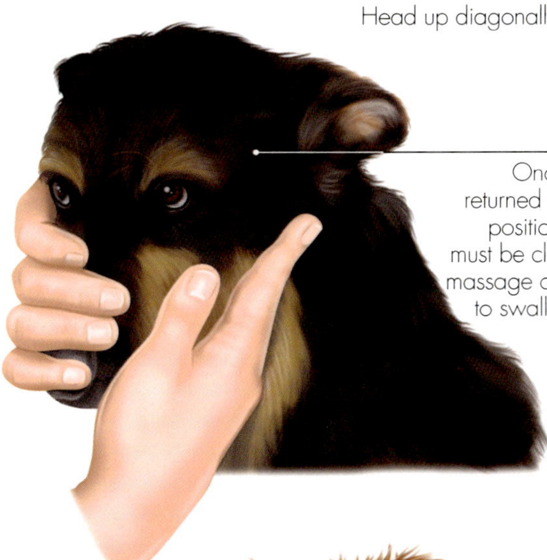

Once the head returned to a normal position, its mouth must be closed and a massage on the throat to swallow is given

Liquids and pastes

The dog's mouth is closed and the tip of the syringe is inserted into the comissure, in the hollow behind the molar teeth

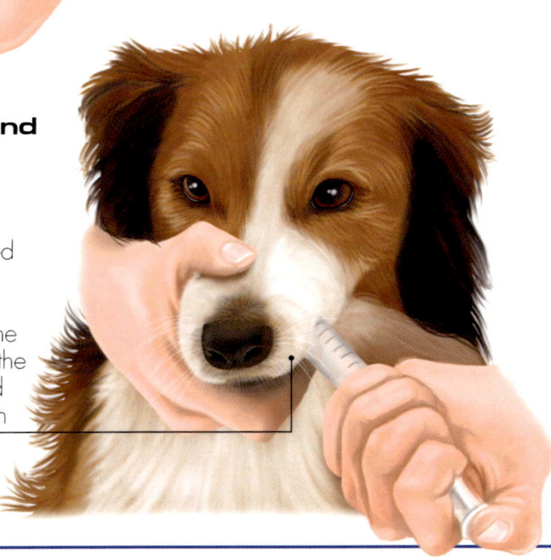

Eye drops

The hand with the eye drops should be supported on the skull so that the drop falls into the eye

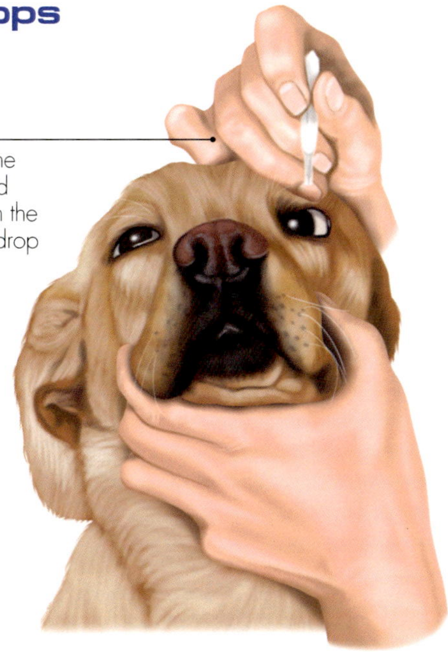

Subcutaneous injection

A great fold of skin must be picked and keep it up while injecting parallel to the dog's body

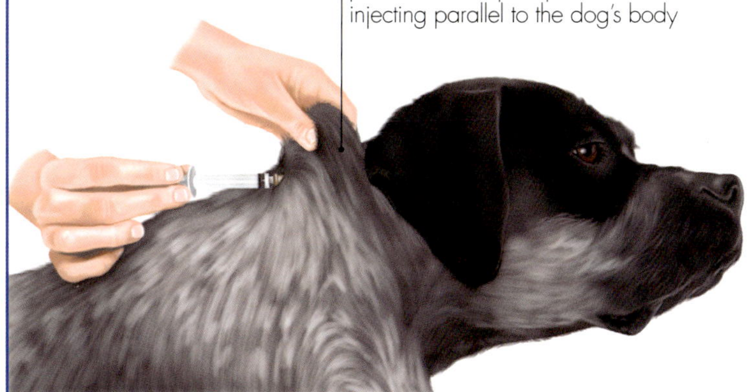

Recommendations

- It is important to show calm and speak softly while drugs are administered, as well as praise them and reward them after that.
- Tablet should not be placed laterally in the mouth, as the chewing reflex is promoted, resulting in rejection.
- Daily walk may be used, as the dog will be more entertaining and easier to "cheat" to take the drug.

68 Reproductive behaviour

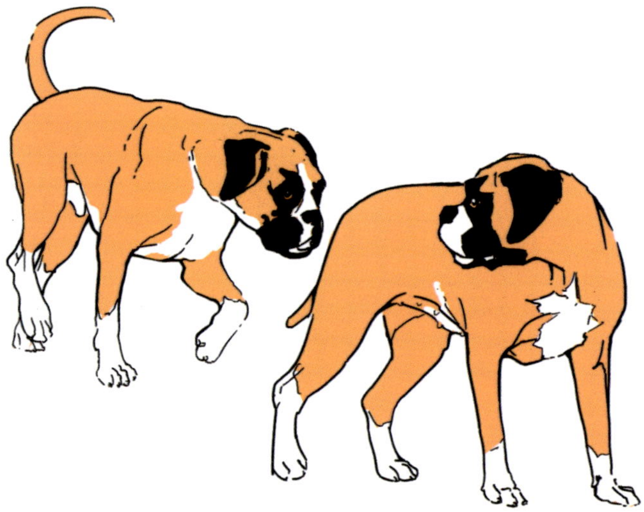

The male sniffs and licks the female's vulva.

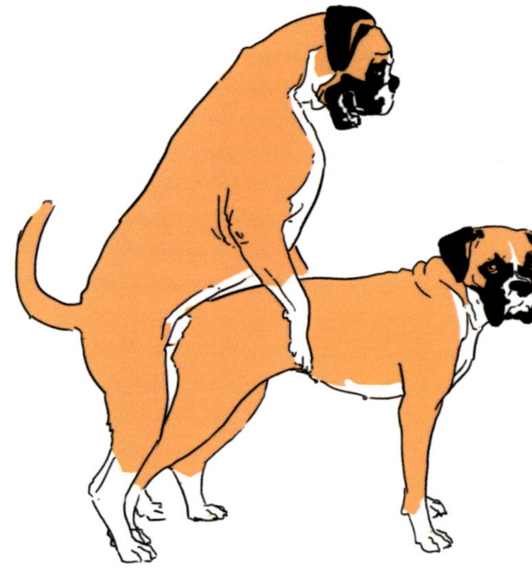

Once excited, mounts on her lumbar area and makes penetration. The erection is passive through the vulvar muscles.

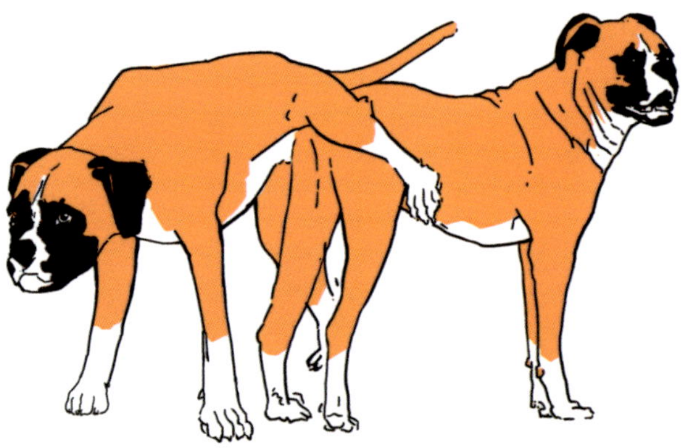

It is very important that the male forms the "knot" inside the female's vagina for the entire ejaculate stay inside.

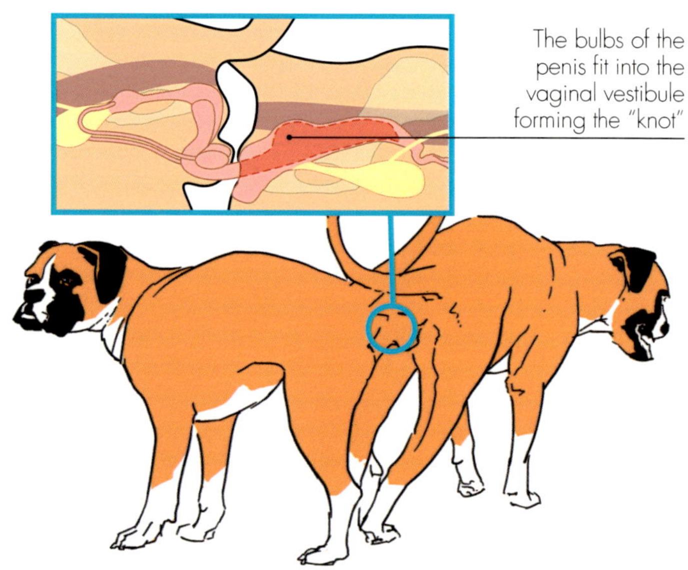

After the ejaculation the female and the male can be coupled oriented in opposite directions even up to an hour.

Getting dog sperm

- Natural breeding must be accurately simulated, preferably outdoors or in a quiet and spacious place.
- The presence of a female in heat helps the extraction and improves the semen quality.
- Press behind the cavernous bulbs to produce the full erection of the penis.
- Let the dog turn around as would naturally occur.
- Semen is collected in a sterile container at about 36 °C. Then, its quality must be assessed under the microscope.

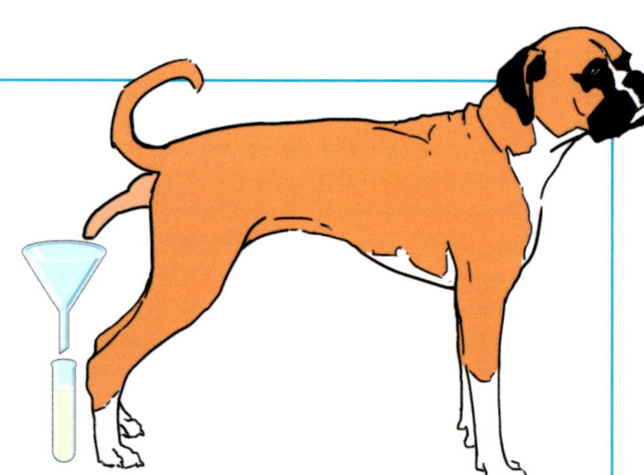

69 Usual postures in dogs

Friendly expressions

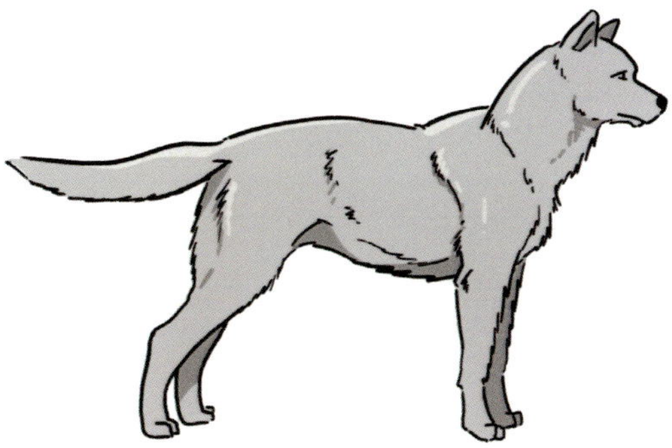
ALERT

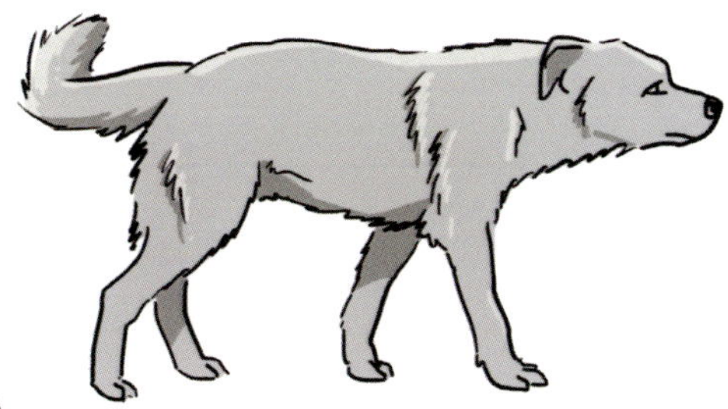
CALM APPROACH

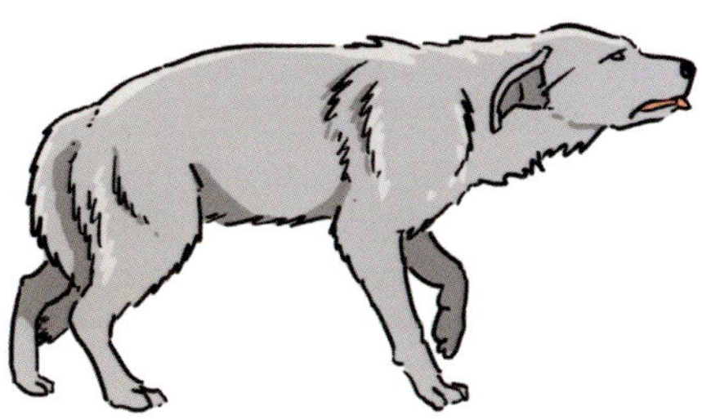
PEACEMAKER APPROACH

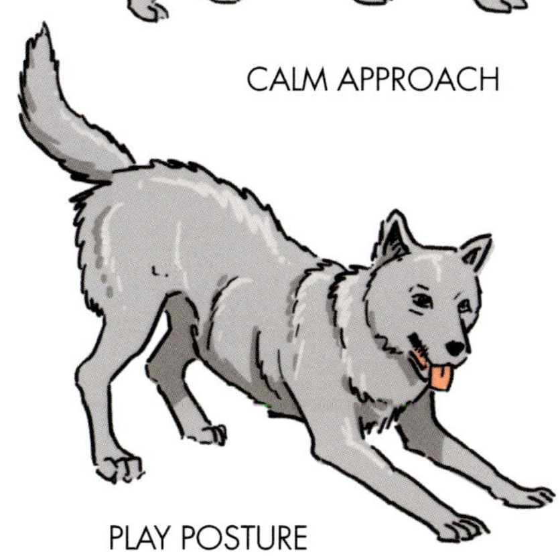
PLAY POSTURE

Aggressive or fear expressions

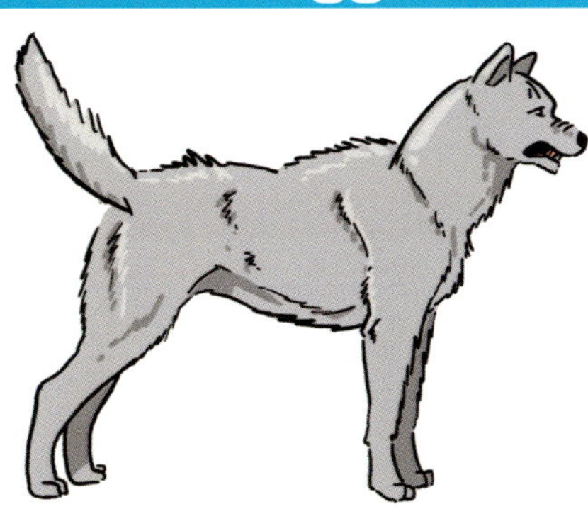
DOMINANT POSTURE

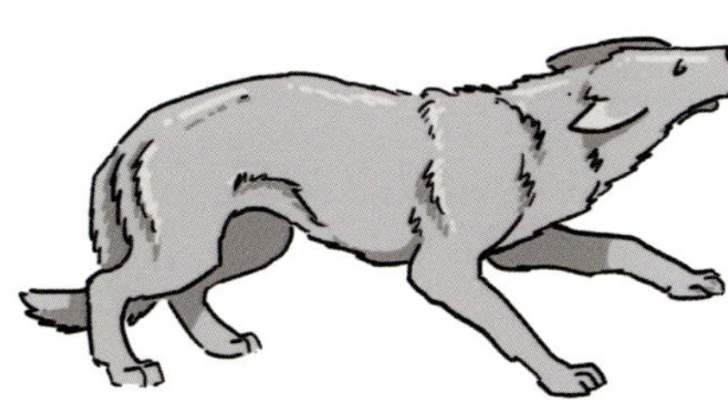
SUBMISSION / FEAR

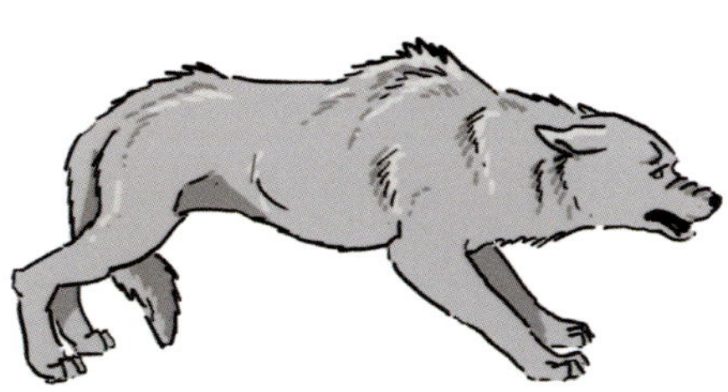
FEAR / AGGRESSION

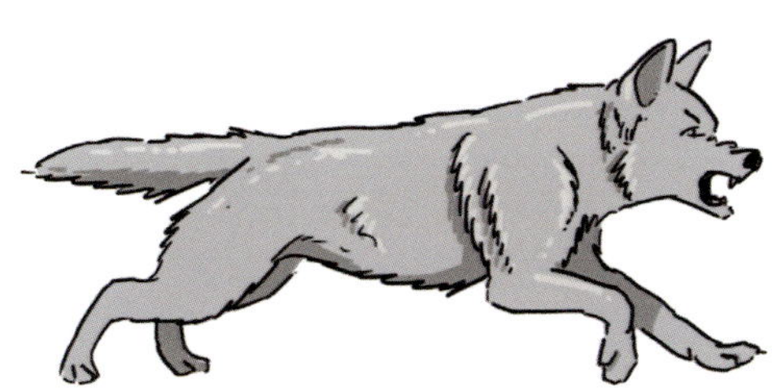
ATTACK

70 Handling and care of newborn puppies

Canine neonatal period encompasses the first two weeks of life. The mother, after birth, is responsible for puppies care and feeding, but if this does not happen, there are some basic care guidelines that should be followed.

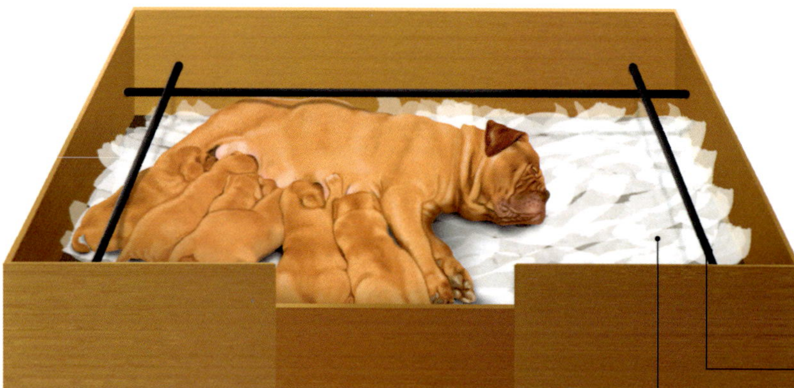

Suitable environment

- Clean and calm, free from drafts.
- Room temperature:
  - First week: 30-32 °C.
  - Second week: 25-27 °C.
  - From the third week: 22 °C.
- Moisture: 60-65 %.

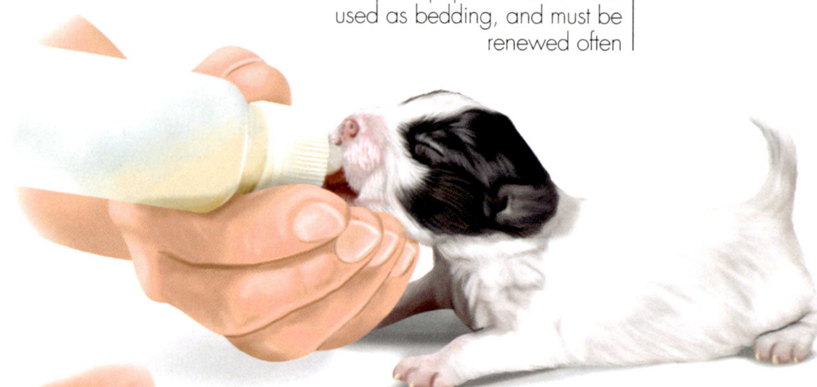

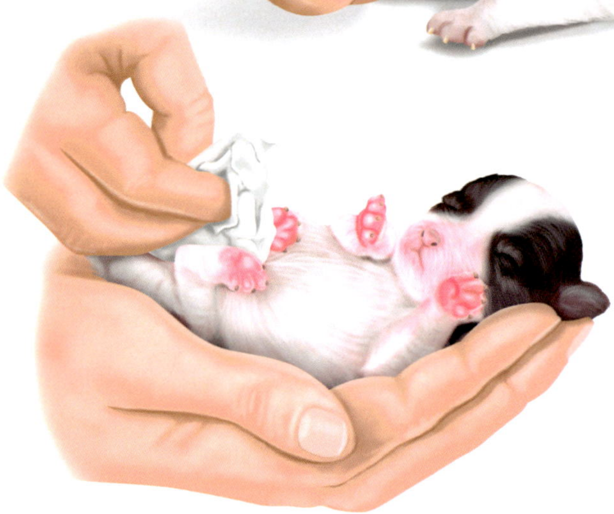

Newborn puppies usually sleep about 20 hours per day and feed during the remaining time.

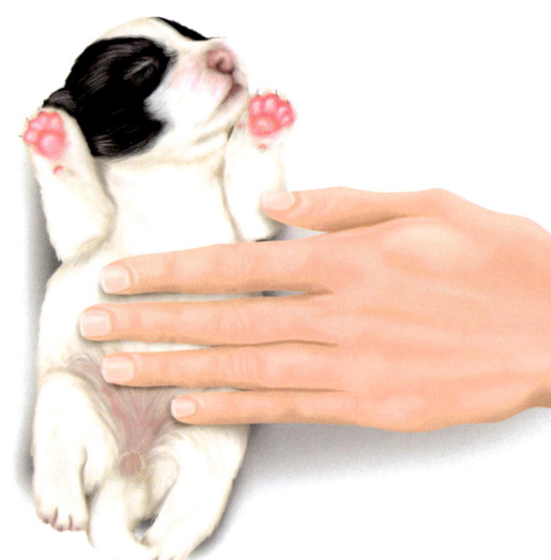

Orphaned puppy care

- The position of the puppy to take the bottle should be like that naturally adopts suckling, with the abdomen resting on a surface or on the carer's hand.
- They should be fed every 3-4 hours (at 35-38 °C).
- The feeding bottle must be washed and sterilised after each use, at least once a day.
- It is necessary to stimulate urination and defecation after food intake through a massage in the perianal area with a warm and moistened swab. At 3 weeks, puppies must do it without help.
- A soft massage on the abdomen should be done at the beginning of the digestion to stimulate it and avoid colic.